"*Health Beyond Medicine* tackles the issues concerning our current medical system. As my personal chiropractor, Dr. Paton helped me restore optimal health through his treatments and return to professional basketball. I recommend this book to anyone who is in search of better health."

—Lawrence Funderburke,
ex-player, NBA, Sacramento Kings and Chicago Bulls

"I love this book! It will help people take responsibility for their health by showing them that there *are* alternatives to the current 'disease care system' in America. Dr. Paton's five factors of health are the means to shift our focus to a true '*health* care' mindset. This book should be required reading for all medical students."

—Jamie M. Schmidt, PA-C

"A must-read for anyone seeking better health. This book is enlightening, informative and life-changing. Dr. Paton's insights and experiences are truly a gift."

—Sara and Corey Kersten, DCs

"The book is thorough and extremely well-referenced, and obviously took a great deal of time and effort. I admire Dr. Paton's dedication to living and teaching the mission. I am impressed, to say the least."

—Dan Roney, DC

"I have been researching health, the history of healing and the methods that have been used for several years. Although much has changed, truth has never gone out of style. Dr. Paton's passion and expression for the truth rings true with every page of this book. We are in an age when, regarding our health, it is time to tell the truth. We will not get it in an advertisement or drug marketing campaign but hopefully, people will take notice of this information and ultimately take responsibility for what is right."

—Timothy Young, DC, FASA

HEALTH BEYOND MEDICINE
A Chiropractic Miracle

Dr. Scott Paton
Doctor of Chiropractic,
Certified Athletic Trainer,
Masters in Sport Injury,
Chiropractor Certified in Acupuncture

Healthcare Unity Press

Book design by:
Arbor Books, Inc.
19 Spear Rd.
Suite 301
Ramsey, NJ 07446
www.arborbooks.com

Printed by Atlas Books
Cover photo by Lifelong Studios

Health Beyond Medicine: A Chiropractic Miracle
Dr. Scott Paton, DC, MS, ATC

1. Title 2. Author 3. Alternative/Natural/Chiropractic Healthcare

Library of Congress Control Number: 2008929425

ISBN 10: 0-9818083-0-1
ISBN 13: 978-0-9818083-0-7

*This book is dedicated to my wife Janice
and three children Tyler, Nicholas and Hannah Rose.
This book is also dedicated to all the people
who discover a healthier lifestyle after reading it.*

TABLE OF CONTENTS

ACKNOWLEDGMENTS

Most of all, my love and gratitude go to my wife, Janice, and my children, Tyler, Nicholas and Hannah Rose, for having patience while I wrote this book over the past three years.

Special thanks to my parents for opening their minds and becoming more receptive to natural healthcare.

Without great teachers and mentors, I surely wouldn't have been as successful as I have been thus far, nor would I have written this book.

A most sincere appreciation goes out to my friend and business consultant, Dr. Steve Hays, who has taught me how to run a successful practice by being a better listener to my patients, treating them with respect, appreciating their time, giving a good service and taking care of myself in the process.

Dr. Richard Rosenkoetter taught me, fresh out of chiropractic college, how to run an honest practice and exposed me to the sports side of chiropractic care.

Dr. Richard Yennie is perhaps one of the most gifted acupuncturists in the world and has a caring heart unlike any other in the field; he is truly a shining star to those willing to learn.

Jason Borton has been both a wonderful patient as well as an excellent personal coach/consultant.

Out of everything I learned from all the gifted professors I had in chiropractic college and the Masters program, I will always remember the first thing Dr. Rod Rutland said in a research class on day one: "Always question authority." I still apply that phrase to my life nearly every day.

I would also like to acknowledge my editors Heidi Connolly and Doreen Michleski for assisting me in getting my message across to help make people's lives healthier.

It has been said that behind every great practice, there is a great office staff. This could not be more true in my office. Thank you Danielle and Jessie. Thank you and thank you again to all the wonderful patients who have given me the opportunity to take care of them and their families. It's been an honor, and I mean that from the bottom of my heart, to be able to treat you all. I wish more people could experience chiropractic or, if not, just sit in the reception area of my office where they could experience for themselves the looks on your faces as you walk in and out. In most cases, other than the first time you came in when you were hurting and feeling desolate, your expressions are usually full of joy and elation.

You are people from all walks of life. Some are college professors, some are oncologists, some are physician assistants, some are CEOs of large corporations, some are bricklayers, some are teachers…the list goes on and on. You've realized what true healthcare is, and I daydream for a brief moment about what the world would be like if more people could discover this healthcare wonder.

You are also open-minded healthcare practitioners in other fields of medicine; the jobs you do are appreciated and I thank you for helping so many people. I know that one day, I or my family may require your services and I'm confident in the most elite acute care services in the world, provided by you in the United States. Thank you, too, for everything you do to encourage your patients to get the help they need.

FOREWORD
Dr. Edward Pearson, MD, ABHM

America is heading into a very interesting, if not turbulent, time over the next few years or longer. Not only is our country's role as the world leader somewhat now in question, but also the financial state of our union and, most importantly, the state of our ailing health and healthcare system are both now seriously in question.

Take, for example, some of the following statistics: The United States is 37th on a list of developed countries for effectiveness of our healthcare system, and this number falls to the 80s when per capita income and expense of the system, or health per dollar spent, is taken into account; our healthcare expenditure makes up nearly 20% of our GDP yet we must ask what we get for all of this expense; and, for the first time in centuries, life expectancies are declining, and death rates for many patient populations, such as birthing mothers, are increasing. These statistics, and many other facets of our so obviously for-profit healthcare system, are passing any point of reason, into a state of unacceptability and even embarrassment.

For those of us in the more natural healthcare fields, as Dr. Paton is, where we are not just searching for the answers but finding them, we can no longer continue to turn a blind eye to the type of healthcare that the majority of people get. For over a century, the major associations of our healthcare system have used fear and scare tactics in the name of 'science' to push all other time-tested and safe, natural healthcare systems under the rug—but no longer.

The masses are asking for answers, and are spending their own hard-earned dollars to receive them.

In the field of what I like to call New Medicine, which is an integration of holistically guided but scientifically based natural healing (*unbiased* science, I should add), we are beginning to see undeniable evidence that the 'paradigm shift' in healthcare that we so badly need is poised to *prove* that a new direction is about to become 'mainstream.' No longer is this 'Complimentary Alternative Medicine'—the future of healthcare and medicine is here, and it will be *the* conventional treatment model within the next few decades. But, it is available now.

I will tell any 'prescription level' practitioner out there that we will still prescribe in the future, but we will prescribe much more natural products to restore health, balance, and vitality to our patients more effectively and quickly than anything possible with today's medications. M.D.s and D.O.s must learn this New Medicine to remain 'the quarterbacks of care' in the more natural healthcare system of the future.

In *Health Beyond Medicine*, Dr. Paton does a wonderful job describing how our healthcare system reached this point, with its foundation based on corporate profits, funded science, and hardcore marketing practices. It is these same practices that now appear to be clawing and gasping for air as big news of adverse effects and corporate scandal within the industry become a common occurrence. Patients are sick and tired of being sick and tired.

Unfortunately, America is no longer the place to be for the best healthcare in the world, not to mention the expense. As always, there is no denying that our technology and progress in 'artificial and synthetic' needs in emergency care and chronic illness management are very advanced. There is no doubt about the skill level, training, and intelligence of today's doctors.

Yet more and more patients are wondering why they are shuttled more and more quickly through assembly line evaluations and procedures only to come out the other end on more medications, at more expense, and more risk. All the while our country becomes undeniably sicker and sicker. Why do today's medical doctors appear only skilled in prescribing medications, disenchanted with their careers, and so unhealthy themselves?

In the aggressive takeover of healthcare by pharmaceutical and surgical methods at the expense of so many other available, useful, more natural, and safer healthcare treatment models, citizens of this country find themselves in a place where many doctors are afraid to practice anything but the 'Western' model.

Adding to this healthcare dilemma, as Dr. Paton has very proficiently explained, is the carefully planned and executed system inducing patient reliance on healthcare insurance, which, again due to the nature of corporate profit seeking, has seen premiums climb astronomically higher while the quality and choice of care is in tremendous decline. In addition, the allowance and ever-increasing number of synthetic chemicals and hormones into our food chain has caused once-rare conditions of chronic illness to increase at truly epidemic rates and to become an 'expected' part of aging...now being seen at much younger ages. This irresponsible technology must stop.

These problems are now so self-evident, so unacceptable in so many and so young, and the industry is fighting so aggressively to maintain its position while more people are simply choosing to spend their own money to visit more natural practitioners such as Dr. Scott Paton (patients flock to his healing treatments by the hundreds daily), that the tide is obviously turning. It will most likely take, as most legally and financially based battles do, years or even a few decades for the tide to shift from the flood of synthetically based treatments fraught with dangerous side effects to the ebb of a treatment system incorporating much more natural (but, in actuality, even more scientific) solutions that are organic in origin, integrated in services, and holistic in scope.

In a phrase, this new healthcare system will be about accurate analysis and evaluation of the 'balance' of health Dr. Paton discusses, not for the purpose of diagnosis of an icd-9 code and prescription of a synthetic drug or procedure, but for the purpose of first educating the patient on the state of their health balance and future risk for 'disease' development, then providing a treatment plan based on naturally restoring balance and, lastly, truly preventing the chronic illness increasing at such alarming rates today.

A text such as *Health Beyond Medicine* should be standard initial reading for our current and future generations to explain the history of where soon-to-be yesterday's American healthcare system went wrong and why, and how it will soon be, in a way, a subspecialty of acute emergency and chronic illness management to be only used in times of dire need when the future healthcare system is unable to naturally restore balance in a body 'too far gone.' In today's system, without this kind of care, most everyone's body is unfortunately heading in that direction.

Fortunately, with the guidance of practitioners such as Dr. Paton, the future of our healthcare system is much, much healthier.

INTRODUCTION

It's not every day that someone like me thinks about writing a book. In fact, I don't know if I ever considered it before my life took a few big turns to lead me into healing and healthcare.

Right up until the time I became a student in chiropractic college, I had a symptom based mentality; if nothing hurt, I was healthy. From the time I became a chiropractic student to now, my view of healthcare has changed almost completely. The more I practiced, the more patients I came in contact with who were thoroughly wasted by disease and despair, never truly addressing the cause of their problems, only covering them up with medications.

The problem has many roots and the solution is not simple. One major problem is the fact that our medical system is corrupt and discourages people from hearing the truth about healthcare. The very trusting American public is being misguided down the same "symptom based" path, year after year. You will wander aimlessly on an endless search if you continue only treating symptoms, and I assure you that you will never find health. You must realize that true health comes from within.

Your body has the ability to function normally, or in balance, allowing you to feel your best. When your body is out of balance, it's time to see a chiropractor. My patients realize this, and it shows. Most people come to my office because they want to feel their best, not to treat pain. Sit in my reception room and you'll see happy, smiling people walking in and out. For those readers who have never been exposed to chiropractic, this is a difficult concept to accept because you're so used to going to the doctor when you feel awful.

You see, you felt awful because you waited too long to get your body back in balance. By getting adjusted, and living a healthy lifestyle, you prevent yourself from even getting to the point of feeling awful. Medicine today has no respect for the importance of promoting balance and harmony within our body. I hope this book begins to change that.

I had never considered that a book of any kind was in my future. I educate my own patients on true healthcare, but I certainly didn't have the time to write a book. That was until a completely life-changing event took place just after the birth of our second child, Nicholas. He had several complications that ultimately put him in the intensive care unit of the hospital. The various paths that the hospital took chasing my child's symptoms, based on blood tests as well as other diagnostic tests, kept leading to dead ends. The final diagnosis was made as a best guess, since all other tests were "normal." Ultimately, it was a chiropractic adjustment that changed my child's life for the better and made me more of a believer in chiropractic than I had ever been.

With so many sick children (and adults) out there, I realized that it was time to show people the truth about healthcare. I absolutely needed to sit down and write a book because of how many other parents have sick children who never seem to get healthy. Now, my children never have sore throats, ear infections, etc. because they get adjusted regularly. I want to share what I have learned so everyone has the opportunity to live as healthy a lifestyle as I, my wife and our children do.

Even though I never expected to write a book, if you'd asked me if I *were* to write one what the topic would be, I guess I would have said sports injuries. After all, I have the credentials of a certified athletic trainer (ATC) and a Masters degree in management of sport injury, so that's one of my specialties. But the road of life often leads us in directions previously unforeseen. The message for me was resoundingly clear and it came in a moment of awakening on the day of my son Nicholas' birth.

The following is the e-mail that I sent to friends and family when my son was released from the hospital several days after he was born.

Dear Friends and Family,

Here's an update on Nicholas. He was born on June 7th by C-section and was doing very well initially. The next day he began spitting up and his lips turned a steely gray/blue. So he was put into pediatric ICU for safety. There he was examined by a pediatric cardiologist, a gastrointestinal doctor, and other specialists. All the doctors (who, by the way, were all very kind, approachable and caring) said everything was great, and that they didn't know what was going on.

By default, they diagnosed him with acid reflux and put him on Prilosec [a drug used for treating acid-induced inflammation and ulcers of the stomach and duodenum] and Tagamet [used in treating certain types of intestinal and stomach ulcers]. But after being on the medication, he had another unexplainable episode of losing his breath, bluing of the lips, etc. So the pediatrician ordered him to stay in the ICU for at least two more days for observation and to hopefully figure out why this was happening.

Janice and I were really stressed out by this point, and not getting the answers we hoped we would. I felt desperate and it came to me that I needed to DO something. I told Janice that I needed to do my part: I needed to adjust our son. I went over to the bassinet and took hold of my son's little body, right there in the ICU. As I made the adjustment I felt two bones in his spine palpably move into place. And, lo and behold, no more episodes of breathing disorders, spitting up, or bluing of the lips. His symptoms went away completely. Nicholas was released shortly afterwards and I am happy to report he is doing well.

We ran into a friend in the hospital while we

were there whose child was born around the same time as Nicholas and who, ironically, had also been admitted to the ICU. His child was suffering from seizures, and his breathing was stopping spontaneously. His doctors told our friends that everything "looked normal" and that they couldn't explain the episodes. As a parent I know just how terrifying this is to hear.

At that time there were a total of forty-nine infants in the ICU while we were there, and I wondered how many had tests suggesting that "everything looked normal." Granted, there are premature infants, those with pneumonia, etc., who need to be nowhere else but the ICU—and God bless the ICU for helping those children. But forty-nine children at the same time???

Our medical system needs to begin to start thinking outside the box, to be more open-minded to alternative treatments and to understand that there are causes to the disorders that arise. The majority of medications out there don't fix anything; they merely mask a symptom so it won't show up in a test.

Anyway, what I am trying to share with you is that you have options. If you know anyone who has children who are sick with constant sore throats, headaches, breathing problems that include bluing of the lips, or any of the other maladies for which the doctor's response is that everything looks "normal" or for whom the symptoms persist despite all conventional treatment, PLEASE send them to a chiropractor. I'm not saying that chiropractors fix everything that comes across their exam tables, but it's safe and noninvasive and absolutely worth a try.

Please don't think that I am knocking medicine. If I break a bone, I won't be visiting a chiropractor or acupuncturist, I'll be seeing an orthopedic surgeon. In this case I'm definitely glad I was in a hospital when my son wasn't breathing properly because if he had

*stopped breathing, the hospital had the equipment to
keep him alive.*

*On the other hand, I am more of a believer in
chiropractic now than I ever have been. And I believe
that this experience has become my "charge" and has
led to my calling.*

I need to write a book.

Love,
Scott

Life

Of the approximately seventy-three to eighty years each of us has on
this Earth, around sixty can be termed the "productive years"
(subtracting early childhood and late stage senior years). That is:
sixty years during which we can go out and have a positive influence
on the world around us. Sixty years of productivity until our last
days, the days just before we become one with the Earth and cease
to exist, at least as physical beings.

It is unfortunate, then, that even with this prior knowledge that
our time is so limited, many of us wander aimlessly through life,
perpetuating close-minded attitudes and being unwilling to
consider different ways of looking at things. Stuck in old ways of
thinking about many facets of life, we're stuck in lives that leave us
frustrated and unhappy.

It is my belief that every one of us should make each of those
sixty or so years the most positive, open-minded and productive
we possibly can. One of the reasons I believe this so strongly is
because I like to think that with that kind of individual commit-
ment on a grand scale, the world would exist in a harmony
previously unknown.

Think of your life as a book. When you're on your deathbed,
would you want to pass on to the next life with a lot of blank pages?
Would you like the spine of the book to remain without a name? Or
would you want to see a title that read *This Person's Glorious Life*, see
a book full of page after page of stories that told of passion and a
fully-lived existence?

Personally, I want to live every day to the fullest so that when I am at the end of my time here on Earth I can look back and know that I did everything I could to contribute in the best way possible to my family, my friends, my community, and the planet at large.

How does this relate to "health beyond medicine"? It's very simple really, because people who live healthier and happier lives are in the position to make that kind of contribution to the world around them, and to help others do the same.

Unfortunately, however, so many of us are not living up to—or even near—our full capacities. Why? Because somewhere along the line we've lost the ability to trust, to live well, and to dream, and somewhere along the line we've lost the purity with which we were born that allows us to live those positive, open and productive lives. And without that ability, we are unhappy, bored, discontent, angry, fearful or depressed , and this unhappiness, boredom, fear, etc. produces an acidic state in our body which leads to illness of all kinds, physical conditions which then lead to more sickness, more disease and longer healing times.

The state of our current world is a reflection of this global sense of unhappiness and it is a sad fact that more and more people are suffering needlessly from being stuck in a mindset and in a health-care system that overmedicates and underutilizes the alternative methods available in the Twenty-First century.

Every day I have patients who come to my office trying to find new ways to feel better, to end the ever-perpetuating loop of doctors, medications, illness and general malaise, patients who are suffering from the side effects of their prescribed multiple medications and are tired of the medical system's revolving door. I hear absolutely appalling stories from people who are on one medication for a specific disorder, and then on six more to attempt to counteract the side effects of that one. Many patients arrive on my doorstep because they are at the end of their rope, both emotionally and physically.

But the purpose of this book is not to malign all Western medicine.

The purpose, instead, is to start to help each of you critically analyze the system's good and bad points—to recognize the not-so-good aspects and praise the better ones. It is also to open the minds and eyes of the general population to the true possibilities of *health*care in the new millennium.

It is my hope that by the time you have completed reading this book, you will understand that medical intervention may not always be the best first line of treatment for the conditions you suffer. There is any number of alternative treatments available, including my own, chiropractic, which can alleviate your suffering and bring health and happiness back into your life.

Doing things backwards

We live in a world where we research cars before we purchase them. We check repair records, crash tests, gas mileage, blue book values, and insurance rates. So why, when we take our children to be treated medically, do we simply hand their lives over to the treating physicians to let them do as they wish? Why do we not ask questions about the treatments and their associated risks? Is it because we feel that asking questions of a medical professional would mean we're questioning his/her credentials or ability to treat us?

It seems to me that we're handling things backwards. It would be like going to a used car lot and letting the salesperson decide what kind of car we should buy, including make, model, year and color, and then paying whatever the sticker price is, and driving off. You'd never do that! You'd be purchasing something without any prior knowledge of its reliability and putting yourself and your family at potentially great risk! How could you feel comfortable not knowing if your children would be safe in this car?

You'd never know unless you empowered yourself by doing the research and making sound choices. That's exactly what I'm asking you to do in relation to your medical and physical decisions.

About the five factors of health

It is my profound hope that as you read this you will keep an open mind, and that you will be able to apply what you read to your own life. If you follow the advice set forth in this book, you will be far less likely to get sick and, if you do experience illness, you will be much more able to fight it off more quickly and easily.

You will learn how to avoid the use of antibiotics, sometimes altogether, for the rest of your life.

You will appreciate the wonder and incredible benefits of sleep. And you will learn how good nutrition, along with exercise and positive living, can change your entire life. This book contains many facts, some theories, and some opinions. It is in no way written to slander or rake medicine (of any kind) over the coals. I firmly believe that most acute conditions are better treated by medical doctors; however, with that said, many of these conditions are treated with medicines that have multiple negative side effects.

A person with a laceration that is bleeding profusely needs sutures; a person with a broken bone may need it set and placed in a cast. When a person suffers a heart attack, or is even diagnosed with cancer, they require some kind of medical treatment. The point is that conditions require treatment, but what kind of treatment is not always a simple question. Sometimes what matters is not how to treat—but how to prevent. And prevention of illness is based on one thing and one thing alone: staying healthy!

There are literally five factors that contribute to ongoing good health: 1) proper nutrition; 2) proper sleep; 3) chiropractic adjustments; 4) a positive mental attitude; and 5) proper exercise. Incorporating all of these factors over time will ensure you have the healthiest, happiest life possible.

Of course, the proof is in the pudding so, you chiropractic nonbelievers, don't worry. It's often the case that we reject what we do not know or what makes us uncomfortable. If the idea of chiropractic raises the skeptic inside you, that's okay. It's okay if you don't believe, because this is not a religion; it's simply a fact. Just ask one of my many patients who include: clinical pharmacologists, medical doctors, plumbers, pharmacists, CEOs, construction workers, accountants, etc.

What I *would* ask you to do is read along and begin to question why you hold the views you do. Are they based on other peoples' opinions or on your own experiences and research? If you are willing to consider these questions honestly, I'd be surprised if you didn't start to come to the realization that there may be many more possibilities for care that you could be tapping into out there, treatments that you've previously disregarded or discarded due to cynicism or closed-mindedness.

For those of you who may have actually heard something negative about chiropractic, or a specific chiropractic professional, again

I ask you to consider the source. Has this person seen a chiropractor him/herself? If not, there is no possible way of holding a valid opinion. Is this person tired, grumpy, dissatisfied with life, or miserable in general? If so, there may be other reasons he/she feels the need to criticize your attempt at opening your mind to healthier options. Is this person letting his or her own propensity for negativity spill over onto your potential well-being? If so, take a closer look at this person. Observe his health. Is he overweight, tired, with a pasty complexion? Is she out of shape, often sick? If so, why in the world would you ask this person about chiropractic, or about any aspect of health care, *especially your own?*

The fact that almost all of my patients have come to believe in chiropractic as a viable alternative to drugs and other invasive treatments is really the only true testament there is.

CHAPTER ONE

HEALTH CARE TODAY: A BROKEN SYSTEM

I. Healthcare in the United States

According to the World Health Organization (WHO), the United States is the thirty-seventh sickest country in the world (*www.who.int/whr/2000/en/annex01_en.pdf*). The American Medical Association (AMA) recently published a study that revealed the staggering statistic that over 200,000 people die each year from what are termed "medical mistakes."

The reality is far worse, however, since most of the data is derived from studies of "hospitalized patients," and those numbers only incorporate people who died *in the hospital*, not those who died before they reached the hospital (Starfield, B. *Is U.S. Health Really The Best In The World? JAMA*, 2000, 284 pg. 483-485). Additionally, the Joint Commission of Health Care Organizations, which operates the database that compiles voluntary reports of medical errors, acknowledges that only a small fraction of the errors that occur are actually reported (www.jointcommission.org).

What does this say about the kind of system we have in the U.S., where we supposedly have access to the best technology, the best doctors and the best care?

It may not make the most fascinating reading material, but when I read WHO's Health Report 2000 (June 21) regarding various countries' total expenditure on health as a percentage of gross domestic product—that is, the percentage of total general government expenditure spent on health—I felt the shock resonate through my whole body.

Of the 191 countries included in the report, the United States spends the second highest percentage of our gross domestic product (15.4%) on health care. Given that fact, one might think we're doing pretty well, right? Wrong! Consider that although Japan ranked forty-seventh, spending not even half the amount (7.8%) we do in the U.S., it ranked *first* for the highest life expectancy. The U.S., in contrast, *ranked only twenty-fourth, behind countries such as Andorra, Monaco, Greece, Singapore, and the United Kingdom* (www.who.int/whr/2000).

So here is my question: How can it be that a country that spends so much on healthcare is still so sick?

Let's try to put this information into some kind of relative perspective. Two hundred thousand people die from medical mistakes each year—more than from auto accidents! That equals seven fully-loaded Boeing 717 jets crashing *every day* for an *entire year*! One plane crash warrants a lot of media coverage and is indeed a terrible tragedy. Yet, the equivalent of seven passenger jets is crashing every single day—right under our noses.

Why don't we know about this appalling, frightening statistic?

Primarily because it is not in the best interest of the medical establishment for us to know. After all, the same doctors who treat us for our maladies are the ones making these "medical mistakes." These are the same doctors who want you to believe that our health-care system is not only the best in the world but beyond reproach; they are the ones prescribing drugs for every conceivable complaint. Is it in their best interest to educate people about preventative care so they can avoid the pitfalls of advanced medical care—or is it in their best interest to appeal to peoples' fears and willingness to "take a pill" rather than change their lifestyles?

Another reason that statistics like these are swept under the rug is one that has me up in arms. The big drug companies (often called Big Pharma) have become huge customers of television and

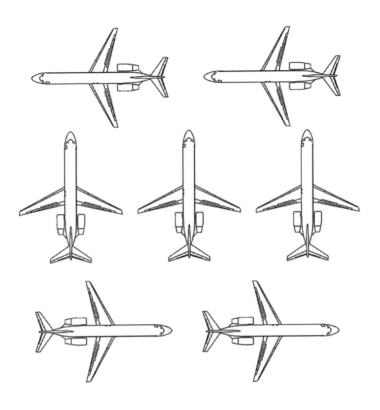

newspapers, paying for a deluge of expensive advertising. This relatively new method of advertising prescription drugs is called "direct-to-consumer" (DTC) advertising and is legal in only two countries, the United States and New Zealand.

Basically, this kind of advertising raises ethical questions as to the psychological effects of seeing ad after ad promoting drugs you "need" and drugs you should "talk to your doctor about, to see if it's right for you" (constantly, by the way, creating new "needs" for seeing your doctor). It also raises questions about our overall healthcare system itself, which continues to focus on treating symptoms, not causes, of all sorts of physical and mental ailments.

Drugs and politics

Advertising like this actually receives quite a bit of attention on Capital Hill. And, while it's true that there are congressional skeptics who claim that DTC advertising is wasteful because it increases already excessive prescription drug costs, these same members of Congress somehow also assert that "DTC advertising is *too effective* because it prompts consumers to pressure their physicians into prescribing unnecessary high-cost 'pioneer' drugs when available generics or the passage of time would be equally therapeutic" (Washington Legal Foundation, 2002).

That's quite a statement in itself, isn't it? First, that the cost of advertising these drugs is what increases their overall cost to people like you and me. But even more interesting is that the advertising is so effective we feel pressured to go to our health care providers to request drugs by name because we "might" have a condition that "might" benefit from this advertised medication.

To me, this kind of advertising is almost subversive in that it encourages people to buy into an inherent need to "have" a condition…to be able to name what you believe, or are told, you have as an illness or disease. In the past we just felt tired, but now we have "chronic fatigue syndrome." In the past we had jumpy legs at night, now we have "restless leg syndrome."

Of course that's not to say that chronic fatigue syndrome and restless leg syndrome do not exist. However, it is to say that there are many potential reasons for these kinds of symptoms and without looking at the total picture—the whole person and his/her history—it's impossible to think that the answer is prescribing a drug (which, in the best case scenario, has multiple side effects, and often does not take the patient's greater physiological status into consideration).

It's also interesting to note that, according to recent studies, people seem to believe that these drug company messages, as commonplace as they have become on television and in print, are helpful in learning more about medical conditions that may affect them (Office of Medical Policy Division of Drug Marketing, Advertising, and Communications, U.S. Food & Drug Administration, *Attitudes and Behaviors Associated with Direct-to-Consumer [DTC] Promotion of Prescription Drugs: Main Survey Results,* available at www.fda.gov, updated by FDA Jan. 11, 2002). Is this because we always had these "afflictions" but never knew what to call them? Or because the more advertising we see, the more convinced we become that we are suffering from certain illnesses in the first place? Or because a symptom from which we suffer now automatically requires a drug to "fix" it—regardless of the side effects that may be incurred? Or perhaps because we believe that drugs are the only viable option for treatment?

In reality, every drug has a side effect, and 218,000 people died last year from them (*JAMA,* 284). In 2003, over one million Americans died from medicine, thus making medicine our nation's *number one killer.*

From 1996 to 2000, Big Pharma spending is estimated to have risen from $791 million to nearly $2.5 billion. Even though that may seem like a lot of money, it is believed to represent only fifteen percent of the total pharmaceutical advertising budget. (We'll talk later about where the other 85% goes.)

Certainly, some arguments *for* prescription drug advertising are potentially valid, but the crux of the matter is that, basically, it was previously illegal to promote drugs on television. However, after a Supreme Court vote under the current Bush administration (April 29, 2002), explicit legal restrictions on DTC advertising of so-called "compounded" drugs have been set aside, citing First Amendment grounds. We have to ask ourselves why such an important issue has been reversed.

We can all see, just by watching a few hours of television or scanning the print media, that drug advertisements are now not only legal, but prolific—and they are having a decided effect on the way we live our lives and approach our healthcare.

Let's talk about the bottom line.

It seems to me that corruption is a natural byproduct when money is exchanging hands in the drug prescription system. After all, if television and newspapers allowed themselves free reign to say what they wanted or to be more critical of the sponsors who hold the economic power, the ensuing bad publicity would cause many of their deep-pocketed advertisers to pull their business. The bottom line is always about the almighty dollar.

Meanwhile, you and I, the consumers, suffer the consequences.

Drugs and television

As recently as a couple of decades ago, consumers didn't know much more than aspirin or Tylenol. We surely did not know the names of prescription drugs and would never have thought to go to our physician to request free drug samples or insist on specific prescriptions. Along with going to the doctor came the understanding that doctors know best—that they were the ones with the knowledge, education, and experience to make the best decisions for us.

All that changed in the '70s when a nightly news show highlighted a specific drug; no sooner had the public heard the news report than they arrived on the doorsteps of their doctors' offices demanding it. It didn't take long for drug companies to get the picture that they could use the media to sell their drugs directly to consumers.

Let's talk about those ads!

On a typical night of television watching, maybe three or four hours for many people, how many drug commercials does the average adult see? With much of television now geared to Baby Boomers, the number of these ads is only going up and it's not uncommon to see three drug commercials in a row (with perhaps one in between about AARP).

It is my opinion that watching commercial after commercial about drugs that are available for every conceivable ill—or perceived ill—is not only a form of brainwashing, but a recipe for disaster.

After all, we are human. Those of us in our prime working years, for example, often come home exhausted from a long day at the office. We want to relax. Huge numbers of us turn on the television for this precise reason. The two screaming children at our feet want our attention, but we're too tired to play, and although we may feel guilty, we're just too exhausted to do anything about it.

Then on comes the first of many commercial breaks. The actor, an unhappy, tired-looking guy, is sitting on the couch—sort of the way you're doing. You can really relate. It's a gray, gloomy day for him, just like it is for you. Now your attention is captured, and you wonder why the guy is so miserable. Maybe he hates his job, too. Then along comes a happy, puffy little cloud with a bright, shining face. The guy is now playing football with his kids and kissing his wife. The dog barks enthusiastically in the background. In lilting tones the narrator tells you that help is on the way, that you can feel happy, less anxious, have more energy, just by asking your doctor about an antidepressant. A voiceover lists the varied and sometimes "rare" fatal problems related to this drug, while you watch people frolicking in the sunshine, on a boat, on a hiking trip, at a party. You don't pay much attention to the voiceover because you're busy being mesmerized by the music or the actors.

I suggest when you see the drug commercial come on, close your eyes through the entire thing. You may be surprised at just how much you've missed even though you've seen that same commercial multiple times.

Just listen to the drug's horrific side effects supplied by the voiceover at the end of the commercial. That's when you are also encouraged to see your doctor—the same doctor who probably knows very little about either depression or the new drug you are now requesting.

So, the next time you hear the words, "Ask your doctor if the pink polka-dot pill is right for you," I suggest you think twice before picking up the phone.

Square pegs into round holes

Another way our healthcare system has faltered is that we've designated "normal" levels for our bodies' substances. We expect that every person should be a circle that fits into a round hole. In reality, some of us are square, some rectangular, and some triangular. Some people have naturally slightly elevated blood pressures, and others have naturally lower blood pressures.

Of course, dangerous levels do exist. When blood pressure is excessively high (when systolic rises above 150 and when diastolic rises above 95 for a consistent amount of time), the situation needs to be addressed, and often when it reaches this point the only way to do it is with medication.

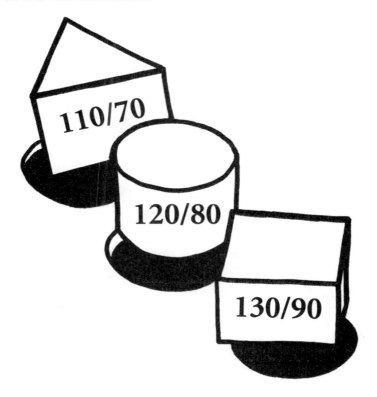

But it is the reason *behind* the excessively high blood pressure or LDL cholesterol that must be addressed. Could it be diet, lack of exercise, lack of sleep, or maybe stress level? Indeed, it could be all of the above. Instead of addressing—or helping patients address—their base cause of symptoms, doctors in the United States keep patients on medication permanently, allowing them to avoid the reasons for the original medical condition.

Lowering blood pressure naturally is often a viable option, but it's not always easy to change our lifestyle accordingly. Telling someone to choose the path to better overall health, so as to avoid having to change this path later on in life, may not be as compelling as we'd hope. On the other hand, when we make the choice to circumvent that path by staying on medication indefinitely, we are also choosing to believe that option does not come with its own set of negative repercussions.

In other words, we are choosing to not see what is right in front of us.

The effects of coercive advertising

We—often knowingly and willingly—take into our bodies things we can only assume will hurt us in the long run. These drugs present an appealing option for handling the vast array of medical difficulties we will eventually face. Dealing as we are now with rampant numbers of ADHD, autism, and childhood obesity, it's obvious that we no longer have to wait for adulthood to experience the repercussions of our decisions.

It would be interesting to hear at the end of a KFC commercial that the additive in their chicken makes it not only addictive but threatening to our health. Would we listen to those words of warning? Perhaps not. Some of us would continue to tune them out, the same way smokers aren't likely to read the warnings on the cigarette pack, and the same way that "potential liver failure" doesn't put us off the drug our doctor has recommended and told us is a reasonable risk to take.

Because so much money for studies comes from drug companies, until that paradigm shifts, we will all be at the mercy of biased research.

These drugs have been "proven safe and effective"

What does it really mean when our doctor recommends a drug and tells us that although there are side effects, they are "worth the risk"? There are literally lists of drugs that have been "tested" and researched and "proven" to be "safe and effective" only to be pulled off the market years later (or sometimes much sooner) due to "new findings" about how the drug has caused birth defects, addiction, infertility, strokes or heart attacks. The only appropriate manner with which to approach a drug is: Don't take it lightly. It can hurt or kill you.

I am the first to admit that sometimes we need a drug if there is no other option. But I have found that it's only rarely that a person, given enough information and support, cannot find another way to deal with the symptoms of a condition. The important thing, again, is to look at the entire person as a whole entity, including lifestyle, genetics, nutritional intake, socioeconomic situation, etc., in order for him or her to stay healthy so illness does not have a chance to infiltrate the body. If and when illness does become apparent, the only way to treat it is to treat the whole person.

The drug company epidemic

The "drug company epidemic" will not be going away any time soon with so much potential profit at risk. Drug companies are well aware that the more we realize the benefits of alternative care, the less we will be driven to treat ourselves with profitable drug therapies.

With so many people employed by Big Pharma, including doctors, scientists, laboratory technicians, researchers, administrators, sales representatives, etc., it is no wonder that there is a tremendous investment in keeping us tied to drug usage as the preferred method of treatment. It is unfortunate, too, from my perspective, that so many doctors and scientists begin their careers with goals of making the world a better place by "finding cures," but soon become lackeys of the drug companies who hold their paychecks.

Medicine sells sickness

It is my belief that most doctors become doctors because they have a drive to heal. It is also my belief, however, that one of the most unfortunate aspects of our culture is that medicine has become less interested in healing than it has in keeping us sick.

In setting up a paradigm of treating illness instead of promoting good health, we have created a breeding ground for wellness through drugs. Staying balanced, i.e., maintaining good health, is also a course that requires visiting "healthcare providers," but not necessarily M.D.s, whose businesses rely on treating what has already gone awry.

I sometimes wonder if our litigious society has forced doctors into a corner that makes them feel compelled to prescribe drugs as a "just in case" action to minimize the potential for malpractice lawsuits.

Even more unfortunate, given the vested interest of the drug companies, the AMA, insurance and lobbyists, and the big money at stake, is that this state of affairs just keeps getting worse. It's not better for you, me or our children, for our families, our friends, or our health. It's better only for the pocketbooks of those who buy into the massive profitability of being included in this huge business sector.

It's simply not possible for drug companies to truly want to find "cures" for diseases when curing them would mean no more drug sales and no more profits. "Treating" a disease with a drug therapy over the lifetime of the patient creates a lifetime of profit. Curing a patient of an illness means no more money!

Our staying sick is the only way for drug companies to survive and thrive. Treating us for sickness is how our doctors have been trained and is how we live our lives…ignoring the signals of imbalance until we can't ignore them any more. Then, we go to doctors whose first course of action is to prescribe a pill—often several pills in order to counteract the side effects of the first ones.

It's not entirely the doctors' fault. We, the consumers, would rather take a pill than rectify our eating habits, pursue chiropractic adjustment and acupuncture treatments, exercise regularly to help regulate our cholesterol levels, etc. We are just as caught in this web of easy fixes and instant gratification as the doctors are.

Addicted to the drug mentality

There are so many ways in which we have undermined our own health even as we have attempted to improve our lives. Many of the things we do today—pollute the environment, manufacture harmful food products, spray pesticides—are things that make us ill in the first place.

Children's asthma is reaching epidemic proportions. Is it because suddenly children are born less capable of breathing than thirty years ago? Of course not. We are breathing air filled with pollutants, right down to the cleansers we use and the air "fresheners" we rely on to cover up "bad" odors all over the house. The chemicals, perfumes, particles and pollutants are, with very few exceptions, inescapable.

Breathing clean air has become a thing of the past. No wonder there's so much asthma!

We start our children early in their addiction to drugs. Almost from birth, many of them are taking drugs for ADD, asthma, ear infections, allergies—allergies brought on and exacerbated by the chemicals we eat and breathe.

Did you know that all new carpeting (except "green" brands) has formaldehyde in it—and that formaldehyde is a highly toxic, known carcinogen? A few of the symptoms of formaldehyde reaction are irritated eyes, nose, throat, and skin, nausea, headaches, nosebleeds, dizziness, memory loss and shortness of breath. And that's just one of the many, many substances we welcome into our homes and into our bodies and our family's bodies—creating lots of business for allergists, pediatricians, primary care physicians and, yes, the drug companies.

Once we receive "treatment" for our symptoms, we need to start treating the side effects, because no drug is without them. And the devastating truth is that it all starts with the drugs we put into our children's bodies at a very early age: the drugs we call "vaccines."

As I will discuss in more depth later, these vaccines do much more harm than good, yet they are touted as saviors. And with advertising taking up the cause, even young girls are promoting vaccines to "guard against" the possibility of future illnesses like cervical cancer.

We have no idea what damage these drugs are doing, what the long-term ramifications will be. As unpopular as this belief may be, I do believe that we are injecting our children with prevalent diseases in the name of keeping them "healthy": diseases like autism (which is now manifested in one out of every 166 children!) and ADHD (Attention Deficit Hyperactivity Disorder), which is considered one of the most well-recognized childhood developmental problems today, afflicting approximately 3% to 5% of school-age children (www.webmd.com, 2007). Even common conditions such as persistent allergies combine to create a continuous flow of business for doctors, insurance companies, drug companies, and all the other ancillary profit centers.

The really sad thing is that there are doctors who would prefer not to run their practices in this fashion, but insurance is virtually destroying the chance for many of them to do otherwise. Many of today's medical offices are owned primarily by business executives whose foremost goal is to make money. Many of the physicians who would like to do things differently find themselves in the position of either having to succumb to the system's directives or sacrifice their practice altogether.

Diagnosis: "medical condition"

Most of what we call "medical conditions" are actually manmade. Why do I say that? Because it's only when a pharmaceutical company discovers a drug to treat it that whatever "it" is becomes a "condition" that must be addressed.

Until specific symptoms are studied by scientists, and until research and tests are done to theorize and confirm, generalized assumptions about those symptoms cannot be made. But the catch22 is that the money necessary for these studies is supplied by the very people who have enormous stakes in the results. To sell a drug, they need to construct an illness for it to treat.

Let's examine this phenomenon relative to chiropractic care. Since drug companies only make money from drugs created to treat named conditions, "conditions" without names do not get attention. In other words, no name…no drug to treat it…no profits. Profits are generated by marketing to doctors, who then prescribe the drugs to their patients. Chiropractors, on the other hand, concern them-selves with one—and only one—important universal disorder called *spinal subluxation.*

Spinal subluxation occurs when a vertebra becomes misaligned, causing pressure to be placed on spinal nerves, which then causes abnormal nerve function (or nerve interference) somewhere in the body. Subluxations are removed by having a chiropractor place his or her hands on the patient to remove this nerve interference through aligning the spine and thus allowing the body to return to a balanced state.

Because no drug company has been able to market a drug that fixes spinal subluxation, there's no money in it as a "condition," so chiropractic care is a threat to the profitability of drug companies.

Though spinal subluxations can be responsible for disorders such as headaches, Irritable Bowel Syndrome, ADHD, and Chronic Fatigue Syndrome, just to name a few, and are successfully treated every day with an all-natural chiropractic approach, the drug companies, major sponsors, and financial contributors to the AMA, in collaboration *with* the AMA, are equally invested in denouncing chiropractic care because alternative therapies detract from their own patient profits. Unfortunately, this prejudice against other methods of treatment starts all the way back in the first days of medical school, where students often receive and incorporate information they know nothing about first-hand.

For instance, we have known about cholesterol for many years. It was actually first identified in solid form in gallstones by François Poulletier de la Salle as early as 1769. But how much did you hear about cholesterol and the dangers of elevated blood cholesterol levels before the "statin" drugs—cholesterol-lowering medications—were discovered? The big cholesterol "problem" as we know it today didn't even exist, whereas now it's not uncommon to be barraged with fear-inducing ads that imply we are ALL at severe risk of heart disease: "Breakthrough Natural Cholesterol Reduction System: 60% of people are at risk. Are YOU?"

Also consider the ad about the new vaccine promoted by teenage girls as a way to *potentially* avoid getting cervical cancer…or the ad about how a blood clot "may go" unidentified and be preparing to strike you down at any moment.

II. Big Pharma

Drugs and side effects

In 1998 an extensive study published in the reputable *Journal of the American Medical Association* (*JAMA*) showed that 106,000 people die each year in American hospitals from medication side effects (Lazarou J; Pomeranz BH; Corey PN. *Incidence of adverse drug reactions in hospitalized patients: a meta-analysis of prospective studies.* *JAMA*, 279(15): 2005). As of 2001, 46% of all Americans took at least one prescription drug a day, and these numbers have been steadily increasing.

The leading adverse reactions against drugs are from: antibiotics (17%); cardiovascular drugs (17%); chemotherapy (15%); analgesics and anti-inflammatory agents (15%).

Our current medical system is intensely reactive, quite literally the opposite of the way Thomas Edison anticipated it would become when he said, "The doctor of the future will give no medicine…" The implication was that by preventing illness, medicine would become unnecessary altogether.

In fact, the world has become more and more dependent on drugs to treat all types of illnesses and conditions. The question is why. How has it come about that we are not interested in staying healthy as much as taking pills to offset conditions—many of which we bring upon ourselves through poor lifestyle decisions? How has it happened that our medical doctors learn a first line of defense of prescribing drugs for treating symptoms instead of looking for the potential causes of those symptoms?

Are doctors too easily influenced by the ease of prescribing pills to cure everything from depression to erectile dysfunction? Have they become pawns of the drug industry that throws billions and billions of dollars into research and marketing?

The answers to these questions may not be simple, and certainly doctors are as unique as patients in terms of approach. Indeed, some physicians have organized to change the way their medical practices handle pressure from drug companies, such as the No Free Lunch initiative, an organization that asks doctors to take a pledge not to receive drug company representatives.

However, certain facts cannot be ignored. For example, we know that for a long time university research laboratories prided themselves on their credibility and objectivity as bastions of independent research. Now Big Pharma money funds many university research studies.

We know that Big Pharma has the money to pay a huge sales force to bring their drug messages to the medical establishment (along with cruise tickets, vacations, and gourmet coffees).

We know that Big Pharma hires laboratories to do their drug research studies with certain specific outcomes in mind, and if the outcomes are not to their liking, they likely terminate that funding.

It's not fair to say that scientists and doctors start their careers aspiring to sell out to the system. But "the system" has the money to fund research. And even the most scrupled medical professionals need to have money to fund their research.

Unfortunately, since so much of the money these days comes from drug companies, the emphasis on healing is on drug therapies, to the distinct disadvantage of so many other potential treatment options. Drugs have become the way, to the detriment of healthcare at large and the health of each of us in particular.

Doctors influenced by the Big Pharma companies, either willingly or relatively unconsciously, have sold out to the system, influenced by the attractive salespeople (called "pharma babes") who provide coffee and a smile, along with the incentive to buy into prescribing drugs, and into prescribing certain brands over others.

New drug after new drug...after new drug

The fact that so many new drugs are released into the marketplace so often is another reason that even a doctor who makes it his/her business to study the various drugs carefully (by reading the research studies in medical journals) would be hard-pressed to keep up with all the new developments.

Take pain medication, for example. The National Center on Addiction and Substance Abuse (CASA) at Columbia University recently published a report titled *Under the Counter: The Diversion and Abuse of Controlled Prescription Drugs in the U.S.*, stating that practitioners are poorly trained in recognizing and managing addiction and treating pain in patients (www.casacolumbia.org/July 2005). The findings were that many prescriptions for pain and psychiatric medications are written by primary care physicians, who typically do not have the specialized training needed for treating such conditions.

According to the report, only 55.4% of the M.D.s surveyed received instruction during medical school in prescribing controlled drugs. Of those, another 55.4% said they had only received a few hours or less and 34.8% said they received more than a few hours of training but not a full course.

Because primary care physicians treat an extremely broad range of health problems, it must be a daunting task to try to study and master the information relevant to all the drugs on the market. Unfortunately, that's one reason the death rate is so high from medical mistakes due to drug interactions. Big Pharma sales reps provide brochures and drug overviews, but how can the doctor possibly know all h/she needs to know before prescribing a particular drug?

III. Generation Medication

Who's to blame?

I refer to Baby Boomers as "Generation Medication" because the term describes them so well. Whenever our children got the sniffles, my mother-in-law was the first to suggest that they get on medication, be it antibiotics, cold medicine, something, anything poured into a spoon and given by mouth. However, since she has seen our children get well naturally many times, she is more trusting that the body has the ability to heal itself without medication.

Nonetheless, it's difficult when you're a young parent attempting to raise your children more naturally, and you have parents or in-laws telling you that they need medicine. You always second-guess yourself. But you just have to tell these family members that you will raise your children the way you see fit.

If they have issues with your decision, restrict the amount of time they have with your kids until they respect your views. Don't worry, it won't take too long for a grandparent to be away from a grandchild before they cave in and accommodate your wishes. Forgive them, love them, just understand that these individuals grew up during a time when medical doctors held answers second only to God's and prescribed a lot of medicine.

I remember my mother taking me to the pediatrician and following his recommendations without question or hesitation. It's possible that things were different then, but now many of the people in whom we place our trust have been tainted by their own learning that drugs are superior to any other method of healing; by their capitulation to the drug companies' coercion; by greed; and by their inability to get out from under the sometimes impossibly demanding nature of providing caring healthcare in a world of lawsuits and mayhem.

Many of the same doctors who went into the field of medicine to heal the sick fell prey to drug companies, enticed into prescribing drugs with lavish vacations and monetary kickbacks. The more they prescribed, the more they received. And that's how an entire generation of prescription drug overuse was born.

It may not end any time soon.

Today, kickbacks are illegal in any form. But the drug companies are smarter than the law. They've figured out a way to circumvent this roadblock by calling their "gifts" (kickbacks) "opportunities for CEUs," which are Continuing Education credits used toward educational goals.

These credits are required by most professional industries to ensure up-to-date knowledge and efforts towards advancement. To maintain licensure, all professional healthcare providers must take career-related educational classes. Of course, classes to enhance learning are always a good idea. But, in reality, what has happened is that drug companies got smart enough to know that sending doctors on unique excursions (which happen to include CEU classes) does not conflict with compliance guidelines.

The compliance guideline issued on September 30, 2002 by the Office of the Inspector General (OIG) of the Department of Health and Human Services states that drug companies can no longer offer money or gifts to physicians for prescribing their drugs. Still, as www.uspharmacist.com notes, pharmaceutical companies put an annual $12 to $15 billion toward marketing to physicians, hoping to influence the doctors' choices at prescription time.

While it is possible that doctors and other health professionals are learning in these CEU classes, it is important to ask *exactly* what they are being taught. How much time is spent during a cruise to Alaska or Hawaii on "influencing the physicians' prescribing choices"?

Given all of this information, it should come as no surprise that more drugs are being prescribed in the U.S. After all, they have been invited into our own homes through television and print ads, and they are thrust into our physicians' offices by the hands of Big Pharma. The question, then, is how do we keep them out?

CHAPTER TWO

DEEPER INSIDE THE HEALTH CARE SYSTEM

Who can we trust?

Big Pharma, the medical establishment, and patients make up a three-pronged force that has contributed to an era of unreliable healthcare and distrust. No one is to blame singularly, nor can we assess the true damages occurring every day.

That's why our only recourse as individuals is to look at things differently. We need to do our research, explore our options, and reconsider previously held (sometimes long-held) beliefs in order to find new ways to handle the care of our bodies and our health.

I also stress that sometimes drugs are indeed the answer in extreme situations. But what I also believe is that the medical profession has lost its credibility as a source for *unbiased opinion* due to pressure from Big Pharma, insurance and, not least of all, its patients—not to mention the difficulties inherent in being in practice, such as the expenses of running an office, medical malpractice insurance, and ongoing education.

I have seen a sad and unfortunate trend taking place in which many doctors have not been able to offset the challenges of the system, at the ultimate expense of a high level of care for their patients.

It is time to seek another system.

Is there hope? The "wellness" industry

The relatively new wellness industry is experiencing a boom. Now that it is projected to be a three trillion-dollar business over the next few years, medical doctors don't want to be left out, so they're changing what they say and do. They used to accuse chiropractors and other practitioners who believed in the validity of natural supplements and treatments of quackery; now, due to the profitability factor, they seem to have changed their tune.

Suddenly "wellness" medical practices are popping up everywhere. To know if your medical doctor is truly wellness based, ask if he think it's necessary that people get checked by a chiropractor. If he says yes, you're probably in the right place. However, unless he is a chiropractor as well as a medical doctor, giving advice on how many treatments you should or shouldn't get means he's merely falling out of wellness mode and back into a symptom based mentality.

If you ask your "wellness" medical doctor if you should see a chiropractor and she responds with, "Why, does your neck or back hurt?" then you're so far from wellness that it's time to find a different doctor. When major economists such as Paul Zane Pilzer make comments about how wellness will be very profitable over the next twenty years, many doctors will unfortunately jump on the bandwagon for a piece of the pie.

Chiropractors have been practicing and preaching wellness for over 100 years, when it wasn't a trillion-dollar industry. We were called "quacks" then. Now that there's a potential for profit, it's suddenly acceptable to find more natural routes toward healthcare.

However, it's not always a reputable route. With medical reimbursements dropping year after year, many doctors are finding additional sources of income through multilevel vitamin sales. They are merely just salesmen in someone else's "down-line," selling overpriced vitamins in their offices. I'm not saying that all multilevel marketing is bad or that all vitamins are overpriced—but selling vitamins out of your office alone certainly doesn't make you a wellness expert.

There is a tremendous difference between achieving health from within (wellness) and masking a symptom. Chiropractic is an integral part of actual healthcare. If it's not included in a "wellness program," then it's not really a wellness program at all—it's just a way to make a quick buck.

Disregarding medical brainwashing, the body knows what it needs to do. We insult it by trying to control it with drugs and surgical interventions, when all it really needs is balance.

Here is a typical scenario:

Two days ago, my two-year-old son got a cold. I don't use the word "sick," which, to me, means there's an infection your body can't fight off on its own. Nick had a cough and fever. We always try to let his body fight it off, let the symptoms run their course by treating them with saline lavages, plenty of fluids, and chiropractic adjustments (all of which will be discussed in later chapters). After a few days at most, he is back to normal.

Unfortunately, most parents, swayed by advertising and medical advice, often react very differently, first with a fever-reducing or cold medicine such as Tylenol. Contrary to popular belief, the illness is prolonged by this kind of approach. Then, after two or three days with less fever (possibly) but no other reduction in symptoms, the parent goes to the pediatrician, who says the child has contracted strep throat or an ear infection. To treat these symptoms, prescribing antibiotics is the only option (this book will go into more detail on how antibiotics weaken the body). Hence, the cycle of perpetuating illness is complete.

An environment has been created in which, because the body has not been allowed to heal itself (with help), bacteria grows into something else altogether. Part of the problem is that from as early as the 1970s, medication use in children has been based on data from studies on *adults!*

I have been accused of being unfair to my child by not giving him cold medicine when he gets a cold. But now there is more and more evidence that treating the usual symptoms of a cough or cold with fever-reducing medications is absolutely the wrong thing to do.

This is 2008. It's been thirty-eight years of putting our children at risk in this way. Pulling the "research shows" card is no longer valid, if it was ever valid in the first place. We have to use a lot more common sense and have a lot less faith in the medical research community.

The *St. Petersburg Times* recently posted an article about an FDA advisory panel's recommendation that over-the-counter cold medications should not be used on children under the age of six. Only a week before this decision, pharmaceutical companies had withdrawn fourteen nonprescription cold medicines for children under two, including Dimetapp, Robitussin and Triaminic—while still insisting that the products were safe at recommended doses. Why, then, I ask, were they taking them off the market?

Though there was no evidence that these medications—all of which were forms of antihistamines, decongestants and anti-tussins—worked for children over the age of six, the FDA panel did not propose restricting their use with this age bracket. The panel did, however, hear from a father whose infant son suffered brain scarring and chronic seizures after taking Dimetapp.

The pediatric branch of the pharmaceutical business includes about 800 cough and cold products and generates $500 million a year. Some alternatives to using these products for a sick child include:

- Using a vaporizer to keep the air moist
- Drying up a runny nose with a solution of saltwater drops
- Clearing up congestion with a rubber nose bulb
- Ensuring that the child gets enough fluids to avoid dehydration—including good old chicken soup
- Consulting a pediatrician—or a chiropractor, for an adjustment that will restore balance throughout the child's system

This is the kind of information that continues to confuse the average parent. On the one hand, the drug industry voluntarily withdrew its products; however, it continues to insist that the drugs are safe and that they work when used as directed.

Unfortunately, when similar articles ask the opinion of the medical establishment on topics such as alternative treatments, they seek information from the same sources, the same "experts," who have provided answers over the last thirty years and who have insisted that these products are safe. The suggestions by the American Academy of Pediatrics are only helpful to a small degree without more specific information. We don't get sick because there is a lack of cold medicine in our body, or because there isn't a humidifier in the room; we got sick because our body is out of balance.

So there are other larger concerns that need to be addressed—in particular, realigning the balance of the entire body so that the immune system can fight off the virus or bacteria with which it has come in contact.

Another case of "it's too late"

When traveling to St. Louis, I picked up the local newspaper, the *St. Louis Post-Dispatch*, and was once again struck by the sorry state of affairs relative to the drugs on the market today.

In the November 11, 2005 edition, an article reported on a popular birth control patch, the manufacturer of which was issuing a warning about increased blood clot risk due to exposure to higher doses of hormones. This, apparently, differed from the information they had previously disclosed. Interestingly, the warning came just four months after the Associated Press had reported that users of this birth control patch had suffered blood clots and even died three times more than women who took birth control pills.

Unfortunately, this was yet another case of too little, too late…too late for all the people who had died and suffered blood clots, too late for their families, and too late to take back the rush to market. It is doubtful that during initial studies, indications for potential problems did not arise. It is doubtful that the drug company manufacturing this patch did not put profits before lives.

"Are our kids the sickest generation?"

Jean Weiss writes for MSN Health & Fitness (www.msn.com, 2007), and, like lots of us—parents and otherwise—is concerned about the fact that more kids than ever before are diagnosed with illnesses such as bipolar disorder, ADHD, allergies, and autism. She wants to know why.

A generation ago most of these problems were almost non-existent. Weiss says that while some people attribute increases to improved diagnosing, and others to over-diagnosing, there are many others who believe that more children are getting sick because they live in an increasingly industrialized and dangerous world—a virtual "chemical soup."

"I do think we are in the midst of an epidemic of these child disorders," says Dr. Kenneth Bock, co-founder of the Rhinebeck Health Center and author of *Healing the New Childhood Epidemics: Autism, ADHD, Asthma, Allergies* (Ballantine Books, 2007). "I don't believe it is all due to better diagnosis."

ADHD is up by 400%. Bipolar disorder is up forty-fold. "Worldwide use of prescriptions to treat ADHD in children has increased by 274 percent, with the United States prescribing more medication for ADHD than any other country," says Weiss. Many children suffer from both disorders. And although the link between environment and illness is more evident in cases of allergies and asthma, scientists are looking harder and longer at links to other types of illnesses.

Dr. Ben Vitiello, a psychiatrist at the National Institute of Mental Health and a leading expert in child and adolescent ADHD, discounts any connection between environmental toxins and ADHD, but there is new research being done which focuses on food additives and their potential contribution to this kind of illness.

Dr. Bock, meanwhile, suggests that cumulative exposure to pollutants (such as heavy metals, chemicals, pesticides, flame retardants, etc.) can increase the toxic load on children who are predisposed to certain medical conditions. His advice to parents? Decrease your children's exposure to toxins by eating pesticide-free food and avoiding heavy metals and harmful pollutants found in products such as toys, computers, and clothing.

"Doctor knows best"

I was recently watching my favorite TV show, *REALsports* on HBO. The episode was about a marathon/triathlon runner named Dick Hoyt, who was considered "one of the best." The reporter indicated that both the father, Dick, and his son, Rick, competed together, but never received different times. How is that possible?

It turns out that this man's son was brain injured when the

umbilical cord wrapped around his neck during the birth process. The father was told in no uncertain terms by physicians that his son would never walk; in fact, he was told that his son would never be capable of much of anything due to the nature of his brain injuries.

While it's true that this man's son is, in fact, incapable of performing athletic challenges on his own because he can't walk, his father refused to take the opinions of the medical professionals as gospel. Instead, he took it upon himself to incorporate his son into his athletic pursuits in a truly unique and inspiring way.

Mr. Hoyt modified his bike to accommodate a space for his son to sit and ride in front of him. During the swimming portion of the triathlon, he pulled his son on a raft behind him. During the running portion, he pushed his son in a cart ahead of him. When Rick was interviewed, he communicated impressively with the aid of a small push button—not with his hands, because he had no control over them. He used his head, the only part of his body he could instruct, to tap the button while he watched on a computer screen to make sure that what he was attempting to communicate was correct.

Even more surprising, though, was that Rick had become fairly self-sufficient. In his twenties, he now lived alone, with a home care-giver to assist him during the day.

Why do I tell you this story?

Because Dick Hoyt has spent the last twenty years *thinking outside the box*. He refused to accept the fatalistic determinations of the medical establishment and, because of his optimism and drive, his son has lived a much happier existence.

So, readers, consider your options first and foremost, and don't let anyone tell you what is—or is not—possible. To learn more about the inspirational story of the Hoyts, visit www.teamhoyt.com.

Is there truth in research?

I was watching *60 Minutes* one day when a segment came on about the possible link between vaccines and autism. The host introduced one of their chief medical correspondents, a man probably in his seventies, and asked him if it was safe to have children vaccinated. The expert's answer was, "Yes, *absolutely*." The chief medical correspondent continued on to say that "research shows" there is (resoundingly) *no link* between thimerosal, a preservative in vaccines, and autism. A similar program aired on NBC's *Meet The Press*.

But the Alliance for Human Research Protection (www.ahrp.org) claimed that the talking heads of television news had been had when it came to the dangers of thimerosal because they had accepted Dr. Feinberg's false claim that the preservative had not been used in infant vaccines since 2003—other than the flu vaccine.

There are several points to be made here. First, information we hear on television from an "expert" (or over coffee from a friend), is not necessarily correct—or in our best interest. Secondly, even when someone, whether it be a chief medical correspondent or a well-respected news anchor, is trying to provide the best information possible, we may not hear what needs to be said. It may not be in the best interest of the people reporting to share the whole truth, or they may be unaware themselves of the complexities of the matter, or the information had not been shared to the degree that the truth could be revealed.

Interpreting research changes results

I've just made the case for why we, as Americans, can no longer take research at face value. If that's true, then on what are we supposed to base our healthcare decisions?

We have always felt confident that we could judge a product on what the "studies show" and what the "research proves," but the only thing we can know for certain in today's world is that someone did some study somewhere that is now helping to promote the product we see in front of us. In other words, it's all about advertising—and the bottom line.

Walk into any grocery store to see examples by the hundreds. Take Cheerios cereal. Its boxes claim that clinical studies have shown that their product can reduce cholesterol, if eaten as part of a heart-healthy diet. And the Cheerios Website (www.cheerios.com) even goes so far as to say that Cheerios is the only cold cereal "proven" to lower cholesterol, citing a study wherein two daily servings for six weeks reduced "bad" cholesterol by four percent. Of course, that was in conjunction with a low-fat, low-cholesterol diet.

Sounds good, doesn't it?

But with what we now know about the kinds of studies performed, how the studies are undertaken, who is paying for them and who is reviewing the results, what can we really know about Cheerios cholesterol-lowering capabilities? General Mills' claim may in fact be true, *but how can we be sure?*

We can't.

Large corporations (like General Mills) have enough money to do as many research studies as they need to, run as many statistics as they can, and design the studies to get the results they want. Even studies submitted to well known journals for "peer review" cannot be considered unbiased because no peer review committee has time for the in-depth analysis required for a definitive judgment.

In *Tainted Truth*, Cynthia Crossen notes that we're all smart enough to be suspicious some of the time, but that largely, we're at the mercy of the companies who feed us the numbers. And we like numbers; we respect them, and we believe them. They help us make complex decisions when we don't have our own experiences or intelligence to rely on. The problem with this is that privately sponsored research, studies and surveys seem to have taken the place of people with actual authority in our lives.

Crossen reminds us that the long history of statistical manipulation that has marked this country stretches as far back as 1840, when the census was basically a fraud, a political tool. She has named the phenomenon of privatized, funded research initiatives "the commercialization of research," a term underscoring the fact that independent voices are dwindling.

Researchers (be they university professors or doctors) can find a way to rationalize what they do and how they do it, but when they're taking money to fund their laboratories or test their drugs, they are necessarily beholden to the funders to some degree. In the medical journal *Lancet*, Michael D. Rawlins noted how difficult it is for doctors to accept that they have been corrupted. They see themselves as untouched by the drug industry but in reality, no one can escape the industry's sales techniques.

It is clear when we look below the surface that even universities are no longer disinterested parties searching for truth. Information and advertising have merged into one amorphous blob that in no way represents an independent evaluation. Research funded privately encourages the tendency to over-report positive results and under-report negative ones.

"Results show"

To understand what this means, we need to define "positive" and "negative" results in the arena of scientific research. "Positive" means only that the results are statistically significant—i.e., not attributable to chance alone. "Negative" means that either nothing happened in the study or that whatever happened could have been due to chance alone.

The goal of the research sponsor is to make their products look good so the emphasis (studies submitted to journals and to the news media, for example) is going to be on "positive" results, potentially ignoring all the other, less rewarding ones.

This is exactly what happened in my research for my master's thesis. When the numbers first came out, the results weren't what I had expected them to be and I was discouraged. I was looking for those positive results, and I wanted to redo the study. But my thesis committee told me it wasn't about getting the results I wanted—it was about learning what the results meant. They insisted that I publish the study "as is," explaining, "It is what it is. Research doesn't always go the way you want it to go."

It is only in retrospect that I realized my committee could afford to be less invested in the results because they weren't being paid by any commercial sponsor. This study was truly independent research that, positive or negative, would have no bearing on profit-making.

In most cases today, however, the research shifts every few years, depending on who's doing it and what results they want. As Crossen notes, there is no "truth" about food that cannot be challenged by research, and that the more a study goes against common wisdom, the more publicity it will get.

To illustrate this point further, Crossen discusses two studies that arrived in the offices of the *New England Journal Of Medicine* in 1986 concerning the effectiveness of amoxicillin, an antibiotic used to treat ear infections in children. Looking at the same data, one study found amoxicillin to be effective, and one didn't. The first study came from a lab that had received $1.6 million in grants from pharmaceutical companies. The other came from a bioengineer who had received nothing for his work.

With so many egregious examples of commercially sponsored research results, it's difficult to choose which ones to list here. Out of the ones Crossen cites, however, a couple stand out above the others:

- The Physicians Committee for Responsible Medicine said (in 1992) that milk was the top health hazard among children, referring to juvenile diabetes. This committee, it turns out, is actually a pressure group that opposes animal research and supports animal welfare groups.
- In a study sponsored by Wonder Bread, the Cooper Institute for Aerobic Research asserted that white bread would not cause weight gain when used as part of a high-fiber diet.
- The Princeton Dental Resource Center suprisingly stated that chocolate could "inhibit cavities." The center is financed by M&M/Mars.
- Back in 1990, "studies" found that disposable diapers were no worse for the environment than cotton ones. Who sponsored these studies? Proctor and Gamble, one of the biggest buyers of research in the United States and the country's largest maker of disposable diapers.

The bottom line is that research can be manipulated with the use of different statistics. There is not just one standardized, accepted method of analyzing data with regard to statistics; there hundreds of totally different ways, each one potentially yielding a different result.

Crossen lets us know in no uncertain terms that traditionally, doctors shielded patients from the "self-interested" pharmaceutical companies but these days, it's hard to tell where physicians' allegiances lie. The drug companies are willing to share their $63-billion-a-year returns with doctors who will do "research" on their drugs—which works out well for some, because with so many researchers competing for support, federal funds have become scarce. Instead of going this traditional route, more and more, doctors and universities are signing far-reaching, multi-million-dollar contracts with drug companies looking for an "official" endorsement of their products' effectiveness.

The major issue here, as Crossen notes, is that this self-interested "research" is the only information consumers may have. It takes thousands of people using a medication over a span of several years to really determine its worth. As Crossen also notes, there's a medical industry joke that says, "Take a new drug when it first comes out, while it's still safe and effective."

To be fair, not all scientists set out to do sloppy studies or be less than objective. In fact, the vast majority does not. Researchers tend to be—or start out—devoted to their professions and objectives, just as most M.D.s do.

There are stories, too, about researchers who have been subject to disciplining and demotion based on their strong adherence to ethics and their choice to place the credibility of their studies over financial offers from commercial sponsors. In one case, though the scientist from a certain university couldn't be fired due to tenure, he was removed as director, stripped of academic responsibilities, his office was forcibly moved from the hospital to the attic of a giant supermarket, and his computer tape of the data from the study was "removed" while he was on vacation.

With the sources that fund scientists, scientists owning equity in pharma stocks, and liberties taken with interpretation of studies to buoy advertising campaigns, results need to be questioned now more than ever—and some researchers themselves agree. Crossen quotes Arnold Kaplan, director of the Center for Biomedical Ethics for the University of Minnesota, who said that if researches are not willing to give up their stocks or their enormous consulting fees, then they shouldn't expect anyone to trust what they say about a drug's effectiveness.

The two sides of research

There is also a critical discrepancy between the two parts of research referenced to make whatever point the speaker is trying to debate: "statistical" research and "clinical" research. Clinical research collects the data, whereas statistical research analyzes it.

In the medical arena, I describe clinical research as brilliant scientists pioneering ideas and theories. Statistical research analyzes the data that was collected when those ideas and theories were tested on people or animals. In my opinion, research gets fouled up when the wrong statistic is chosen to decipher the data collected from clinical research.

Overall, in statistical testing, the larger the sample size, the smaller an observed difference has to be in order to be statistically significant. And the smaller the sample size, the larger an observed difference would have to be in order to be statistically significant. Perhaps the biggest problem is that there's no standardization for choosing statistics, and there are hundreds, if not thousands, of different statistics that could be utilized to analyze the data. Each statistic could potentially yield a different result.

What all this means is that there is a big difference between the two parts of research, and which research results make it into our hands is based more on who's doing the promoting—drug companies, doctors, scientists, or corporations such as General Mills.

Do you remember Vioxx? It was touted as a wonder drug to help decrease arthritis pain without causing stomach damage. Before the FDA allowed this drug to go on the market, they had to perform "clinical research" to make sure it was "safe." Statistical research was performed on the age group most affected by arthritis, our seniors, and brought to market.

Shortly after Vioxx was firmly established in the marketplace as a viable option for treating arthritis, it was found to cause strokes and heart attacks for many of the people who used it. Was this research new? Did the drug company that created Vioxx suddenly discover there were problems? Or did they rush the drug to market without utilizing the proper *statistical research* to ensure the public's safety?

We may never know whether the company that created Vioxx

purposefully released this drug knowing its potential dangers, or if they chose to ignore possible warning signs in their research. We hope neither. But since this occurrence is becoming more and more prevalent—drugs that are "safe" today are found to be highly risky tomorrow—we have to assume somewhere along the line oversights are taking place.

Shortly after I wrote this section, an email arrived in my inbox on this very topic. The story went like this:

Vioxx researchers, it is alleged, had concealed pertinent information—life-saving information—from their study. Approved by the U.S. Food and Drug Administration in 1999, and used by about 20 million Americans, Vioxx was withdrawn from the market in 2004 by drug maker Merck & Co. after a study showed that the painkiller doubled the risk of heart problems. Allegedly, certain company administrators (higher up than the researchers) authorized this cover-up.

Findings of the study in question have been a key part of testimony in the three product liability trials to date over the withdrawn drug, including one deliberated by a federal jury in Texas. Expensive? You bet! One article on this topic went on to say that the manufacturer of Vioxx is currently facing potential lawsuits totaling 50 billion dollars.

Let's return now to our initial discussion about our chief medical correspondent's point of view on *60 Minutes* regarding vaccines and autism. In light of the above information, how likely is it that this statement, "Research shows there is *no link* between thimerosal and autism" can be trusted?

Let's go one step further and look at a possible motive the television industry might have to support the research, however indirectly. While it's true that programs such as *Meet The Press* and *60 Minutes* may attempt to get to the root of the stories they present and show both sides of the issue fairly, in this case of drugs and the marketplace, there's very little possibility of finding the "truth." Even a "medical expert" can be misinformed if the research is biased.

In the case of Vioxx, for example, the corresponding study was published in *The New England Journal of Medicine* in November

2000 before the deception was discovered, according to the *Journal*'s editors. And although the editors "first became aware of the missing data in 2001, they did not suspect any wrongdoing at the time. 'Until the end of November 2005, we believed these were late events that were not known to the authors in time to be included in the article published in the *Journal* on Nov. 23, 2000,'" they wrote" (Alexis Black, www.newstarget.com).

What can we learn from this debacle? That even the most well-versed individuals can misconstrue data—purposefully or not. And when drug companies pay television stations exorbitant amounts of money to market their drugs and are, in fact, *sponsors* of the very shows which may be questioning their ethics or research claims, the truth may never be accessed. Sponsors pay the salaries of everyone associated with the corresponding shows, or other shows on the same network. Therefore, it has to be virtually impossible for anyone related in any way whatsoever to the show or its commercials, its promoters or, yes, even its medical correspondent to stay objective enough to provide an unbiased perspective.

Doctors also have a stake in the outcome. They want to help their patients. They want the drugs to work. They stay current on the research by reading their journals and going to conventions (which are often hosted by drug companies). How is it possible that the "research" results would go unaffected by all the people invested in making the drugs and bringing them to market?

In my estimation, it's not.

Please visit the web site www.drugrecalls.com to take a look at drugs that had to be pulled off the market for life-threatening side effects and that *research* initially indicated were safe. It's extremely alarming to see how many drugs people commonly take can be so life-threatening. But research initially suggested they were safe, right?

The experts "know best"

I'd like to go back to that time in the hospital with our newborn, Nicholas. My wife and I were no different from most parents, trying to do the right thing, believing that the "experts" knew best. Our instincts told us that prescribing drugs for an infant wasn't the best way to go about fixing the problem, but we didn't know what else to do. So we listened to the doctors and let them do their jobs.

Every specialist in the hospital who saw our baby told us that the tests came out normal and they had no explanation why his lips were turning blue and he was losing oxygen. They subjected Nick to what turned out to be unnecessary x-rays (at least five of them— and subjecting an infant to the ionizing radiation of x-rays is never a good thing). Although "research showed" for years and years that x-rays were "safe" in "reasonable" amounts, now we know that each and every x-ray lowers the body's resistance to potentially negative effects from radiation, especially for infants. In the case of infants whose cells are replicating at extremely high rates, ionizing radiation (x-ray) can be dangerous—the same reason we try to avoid x-rays of women who are pregnant.

Yet another example of health and safety concerns arose when our son Tyler was one- year old. We told the pediatrician that we were not sure we wanted him to receive the rotavirus vaccine because we felt it was unsafe. The pediatrician's response was, "But it's safe, it's been researched. And furthermore, if you choose not to get it, we can't treat him. That's our policy."

As you'll read later on, the American Association for Health Freedom recently learned of a family pediatrician who is charging a $20-per-child fee (referred to as an "aggravation" charge to the parent) for refusing vaccines. This is also being applied to parents who question vaccines, want to delay them, or spread them out over time.

Our response was to leave that pediatrician and find another one who would be a lot more receptive to our needs and concerns. And we were not surprised when shortly thereafter the rotavirus vaccine *was pulled off the market!* It was killing babies by causing something called intussusception, which occurs when one portion of the bowel slides into the next, creating an obstruction in the bowel with the walls of the intestines pressing against one another. Intussusception leads to swelling, inflammation and decreased blood flow to the intestines involved. Those babies who don't die from this tend to go on to have painful conditions such as Crohn's disease or ulcerative colitis.

When I learned how close we had come to risking our baby's health, I was really shaken. Later, I researched this vaccine myself and was not surprised to learn that the company that produced it lost their lawsuit in court, and was ordered to pay in the many billions to help offset the cost to all the parents of those children permanently disabled from that harmful vaccine.

What's the alternative?

What can we do? First and foremost, we need to empower ourselves to do our own research, open our minds to examine the source behind the declarations of "safe" or "research says" or "don't worry, the doctor knows best..." We need to make the most educated and well thought-out decisions we can for our own and our family's health.

Secondly, we can consider alternatives. If your doctor had suggested Vioxx (the most popular arthritis drug there was) *before they recalled the drug,* a lack of interest in researching other possibilities combined with the doctors' willingness to let drugs be the solution could have left you wide open for stroke and heart disease. On the other hand, you could have considered a safer, less invasive, less risky course of therapy. Perhaps this course would not be as "easy" as taking a pill, or letting the doctor tell you what's best, but it could have changed your life for the better and for the long term.

Remember, I am also a medical professional, and medicine, per se, is certainly a good thing. In fact, it can be critical in emergency situations. But if there's a problem that might be fixed naturally, why not give it a try?

CHAPTER THREE

EXAMINING THE INSURANCE INDUSTRY

Insurance and the healthcare system

Where does the insurance industry fit into our discussion about the state of health care in the U.S., in our doctors' offices, and in our health?

Notwithstanding all the medical professionals who continue to provide the very best care they can to their patients, there are just as many who have capitulated to the insurance companies. As if that weren't enough, medical doctors themselves have begun to suffer now, too, for having supported the very companies that are now putting them out of business with their low reimbursements.

I see medical doctors practicing out of grocery store chains in 800-square-foot "offices" to make ends meet. Twenty years ago this would not have been possible. The same thing has happened to pharmacists to the point where there are very few individually owned pharmacies left.

When the AMA agreed to reimbursement caps, "in-network" and "out-of-network" physicians, etc., they failed to see how detrimental it would be to their own practices and patients. Where has the noble profession of being a physician gone? There is no such thing as the neighborhood family physician anymore. People are constantly changing from physician to physician due to insurance considerations, and smart medical doctors are leaving the insurance company networks altogether.

Things are indeed falling apart.

Because the situation has gotten so severe, my office now has no link to HMOs because I will not let an insurance company dictate how I treat my patients. When I bought my office equipment it was from a medical physician leaving his practice. When I asked why he was shutting his doors, he said flat out, "HMOs put me out of business. Their reimbursements were so bad I couldn't even make my overhead."

The dilemma

We are in the middle of a huge dilemma regarding healthcare in America. Health insurance companies are thriving and the insurance company's clients (you and I) are suffering. The more I hear from my own patients and colleagues, some in medicine and some in chiropractic, the more horrified I am. Insurance companies are charging exorbitant rates and the victims that fall prey to this scam are middle- and lower-middle-class citizens.

A friend of mine, a medical doctor in Atlanta, called me one day to express just how irritated he was. He was usually a happy-go-lucky kind of guy, intelligent with a good bedside manner to match, so I was surprised to hear him so distressed. When I asked why, he responded that he suspected a patient of having cancer, and had attempted to order a test to verify his findings. He had just heard that the patient's insurance company refused to approve the test. They indicated that there "wasn't enough evidence" to support the test and that the patient would have to pay for it with his own money if he wanted it done.

My friend, the doctor, was certain that the patient did have cancer and needed this test to support his theory. Since the cost would have been much more than the patient's co-pay, he—not surprisingly—didn't want to get the test, and ultimately did not. In the end, my friend continued to grapple with the ethical medical dilemma in which he found himself—wanting to do the best he could for his patient, but not having the means to do so.

He told me, "This patient has paid for his insurance for years. What is it doing for him now, in his time of need?"

I had no answer for him.

I've had the same experiences in my practice. As I said, I will not sign anything that qualifies me as an "in network" provider with an HMO. I gladly accept any patient, even if they are on an HMO that I am not contracted with. I am currently on one major HMO plan, but have been on this plan long before I learned about the insurance truths. When I originally got on this one HMO's plan (when I first got out of chiropractic college) as a preferred provider, a company I'll call "Insurance Company X" was an excellent, doctor-friendly plan to be on. Then, a third-party provider took over all of the chiropractic claims. I'll call the third-party company "XYZ" and when Insurance Company X hired them to manage all of the chiropractic, podiatric, and physical therapy claims, they promised not to undermine the doctors' treatment or get involved in the treatment of the patients.

In actuality, the opposite has occurred. At times the company has sent me belligerent, threatening letters, telling me that some of my patients have been treated with too many visits. They added a warning that if I kept treating patients with the same frequency, I could no longer be a provider on their plan. To this day, I'm surprised that I haven't been kicked off the panel because I haven't conformed to their changes.

During the time I wrote this book, I have decided to fire the insurance company that represented the one major HMO that I was on. I was tired of listening to high school graduates who took a weekend class on how to deny insurance claims try to tell me how to practice. Writing the letter informing the insurance company that I would no longer be a participating provider was very liberating. I highly recommend that all healthcare professionals fire any HMO that they're on. Eventually insurance companies will get the picture that doctors need to be doctors when enough of them leave. You can have very successful practices by being an out of network provider.

In the past, XYZ used patient forms to determine how much treatment the patient would be allowed to have. Currently, they compare all of the doctors' treatments with each other and come up with a statistic called "standard deviation."

To explain, using the insurance example, the insurance company comes up with an average (mean) number of visits that they claim should be enough for a doctor to be able to fix a problem, such as low back pain. The number is usually so low that it's absurd; remember, though, they're putting their investors' best interests first and your health second. The standard deviation is measured in increments (one, two, three standard deviations) from the mean. So, let's say for low back pain, the insurance company states it should take 10 treatments to resolve. One standard deviation from the mean might be two treatments, two standard deviations would be four treatments, etc.

So, using our example, one standard deviation would be 10 treatments +/- 2 treatments, meaning if the doctor sees the patient for 8-12 treatments (10-2 = 8, and 10+2 = 12), he "flies under the insurance company radar." Let's say the doctor successfully treats the patient but it takes 15 treatments. The doctor would start getting calls from the insurance company stating he's going beyond one standard deviation (two treatments) from the average expected number of visits (ten treatments). If he keeps this up, they'll threaten to kick him off the in-network panel.

Some doctors unfortunately give in to these scare tactics and treat the patient less than what is required, so as not to face the ramifications of the insurance company. If you think this is limited to chiropractic, think again. What's terrifying is that it is occurring with doctors such as oncologists, who are treating patients with cancer.

This problem goes far beyond HMOs. A few of my patients have PPOs. With a PPO, you supposedly get more freedom to see whatever doctor you want to see. The only difference is that if the patient goes to a doctor who is not in the insurance company's network, he has to pay out of pocket up to his deductible (which is usually $250, $500, $1,000, $5,000, or $10,000). Once this deductible is met, the patient usually pays a co-pay of 20%, or sometimes 40%, each visit.

The worst part is that some insurance companies only allow a certain number of doctors on the plan to provide care for their insured *in the area where the patient lives*. One huge insurance company only allows one chiropractor on their panel for half the county where I practice. Let's call that chiropractor Dr. X.

Every chiropractor other than Dr. X is considered "out of network." That means patients who choose to have the "co-pay mentality" must drive to see Dr. X, even if they've been referred to Dr. Y by a friend or family member. If the patient has an HMO, his two choices are to either see Dr. X and pay his co-pay or go see Dr. Y, whom he wanted to see, and pay cash for the visit from his own pocket (and no insurance involvement whatsoever).

One problem is that the insurance company makes Dr. X fill out significant amounts of paperwork and cuts the doctor's reimbursement check to sometimes one-fifth of what his or her services are actually worth. But worst of all, the insurance company caps the patient's visits to a maximum—even if the contract states that the insured person gets twenty visits per year, the insurance company could cut off treatments at, say, eight for a specific condition such as neck pain, stating that further treatments are not medically necessary. The insurance company is indirectly treating the patient by placing these limitations.

If that has your dander up, this will push you over the edge.

I recently saw a patient who had a major insurance company's PPO plan, which stated a $500 deductible and 20-visit maximum. The discrepancy is in the fact that the plan had a maximum dollar amount of $750, including the $500 the patient would pay out of pocket towards the deductible!

When the first chiropractic visit is included in the overall care program (exam and x-rays), a $750 maximum may allow for six chiropractic visits. But, at that point, the maximum of $750 has already been exceeded. The insurance company had indicated that the insured would receive 20 visits but, in fact, the patient will never see fourteen of those!

A PATIENT'S STORY

> *I got a notice from my United Health Care (ATM) that said they were no longer going to cover any visits with Dr. Paton. So I questioned whether I had used up all my allocated visits. I found out that wasn't the case. It wasn't that I had used up my visits, it was that they had decided arbitrarily that there was nothing wrong with me anymore and that they*

would not treat me for preventative care. All along, I filled out the forms saying preventative care, preventative care, and it had never been questioned before.

Over the last four months I found out that an oncologist who is treating my friend has been strong-armed by United Health Care and was told that he would have to take less money per office visit. My holistic integrated medical doctor was told the same thing. My ophthalmologist also. And now it's you [referring to Dr. Paton]. It's time for consumers to get involved and tell them that if they are not going to provide good health care for us then things have to change. Providers are just the middlemen really and have to deal with this kind of thing. I'm actually working with someone to get something created for integrated holistic care, which would include chiropractic care. It's wrong for them to dictate what I can and can't do, what I can and can't get done—in a lab or in an office. Fortunately, we've been in a position where we've been able to pay a bit more out of our pocket.

What about all those people who can't?

Insurance for catastrophes

Insurance was originally intended for catastrophes. At one point, health insurance was specifically designated to assist those who were in catastrophic car accidents, who had falls or broken bones...in other words, true emergencies. Somehow, somewhere along the line, it deviated to from that path to becoming a "necessity" for daily healthcare.

We have adopted this "co-pay mentality" to our health, and it is this mentality that has shifted our thinking from prevention to reaction. We react when we feel a symptom instead of trying to prevent the symptom from occurring in the first place. Why? Often because we believe we have that safety net called "insurance." But that "safety net" is why the majority of Americans are overweight, sick, and on permanent drug regimens.

Automobile insurance was also born from the same concept. It was designed to help us with critical situations monetarily and medically. To this day, we don't use our car insurance for the daily maintenance of our car. When our car is making an abnormal sound, we have the mechanic diagnose the problem and fix it. We never ask if it's covered by our insurance.

What about scheduled maintenance? When we bring our car in to get the brakes replaced, we do so to prevent a major, more expensive problem from occurring. If we didn't do this, the brakes would wear thin to the point of doing significant damage to the actual brake system itself. If you think about it, we treat our cars better than we treat ourselves.

Our mentality with regards to our own health care is to ignore the symptoms by taking drugs that cover them up. Rather than go for preventive maintenance (chiropractic, yoga, acupuncture, personal training, nutritionists), we wait for our symptoms to get bad enough that we have to have radical intervention that often doesn't work anyway.

Just imagine how healthy our society would be if we treated our bodies with the same devotion and prevention mentality as we did our cars. My personal opinion on insurance is that your insurance premium should reflect your health. If I work hard at taking care of myself by practicing the five factors of health—eating right, exercising, sleeping enough, getting adjusted and staying positive—I should have no business paying a higher premium to offset increased medical bills from sedentary people who don't exercise and eat cookies all day.

It's a personal choice to look good, feel good, have a healthy weight and BMI (body mass index), and to get up off of the couch to exercise when I might feel tired that day. But I truly feel that I and every other person who puts an effort into being healthy should be rewarded with lower premiums because we won't need to use the insurance as much as people who don't.

The real story behind insurance: an interview

Dictionary.com defines insurance as "the act, system, or business of insuring property, life, one's person, etc., against loss or harm arising in specified contingencies, as fire, accident, death, disablement, or the like, in consideration of a payment proportionate to the risk involved."

Basically, insurance companies like to sell us what they call peace of mind, the idea that if/when something happens, we will be made whole again. That is according to the terms they put in our contract. And therein lies the rub, because contracts have become difficult to understand, full of supplements, caveats, appendages, and exclusions.

Instead of "if we get hurt, we will get the care we need," our insurance companies tell us we will only get certain care at certain times from certain people and to a certain extent…excluding all else. It is the unfortunate reality that if our body is ill, the last thing we can achieve from our insurance company is true "peace of mind."

Many of us don't fully research our insurance companies prior to signing contracts that could significantly, sometimes drastically, affect our lives. We trust the words of the insurance representatives with little consideration for the small print lodged in our contracts and agreements. Some of us believe we are "covered" because we are members of a group insurance plan, but know very little about the plan until we need it. It's then that we find out that coverage can mean a lot less than we bargained for, with prescribed number of treatments, prescribed types of treatment and "pre-existing conditions" for which treatment is not an option.

Because insurance is such a big topic of concern to so many people, I interviewed a colleague to provide some answers to my questions. I'll refer to him with the fictitious name of "Mike Thomas." Mike has been a dedicated insurance professional for many years, working at one of the biggest insurance providers in the country. What follows is the edited version of our two-hour discussion:

DR. PATON: *I'm concerned about many aspects of the healthcare system in the U.S. and particularly about the way insurance companies affect a practitioner's ability to treat their patients. For example, HMOs tell doctors how to do their jobs. A doctor might make the determination to see a patient a minimum of five or ten treatments, for example, and the insurance company denies the request, cutting off treatment after an arbitrary number of times. This is not just happening in chiropractic, of course, but in all fields across the medical spectrum. The other major concern I have is that patients have become consumed by* *what I call the "co-pay mentality"—"If it's not covered by my co-pay, I don't want the treatment."*

MT: Well, Scott, your concerns are understandable. I'd like to start with an explanation of how HMOs work to clarify some of the issues. HMOs are a little different from other types of insurance companies. HMOs are "managed care," which means you're accepting the insurance company's—or the doctor's—decisions about your care. The whole system is a "health-maintenance organization," organized and designed to run through your one primary doctor. If you go out of the HMO to someone or for something that is not "pre-certified," you're going to pay a lot out your pocket. That's the reason many people have steered away from HMOs over the last decade. And there are reasons for concern.

But there are also valid concerns about "universal healthcare" and how a system like that would actually work. For example, there is currently a two- to four-year wait in Canada for finding a primary care physician. On the other hand, the doctors in England provide relatively good care because they get bonuses from the government for having their patients reach certain goals (like lowering cholesterol, losing weight, getting into better health), which eventually helps lower overall health costs of the entire country. They offer doctors incentives to give their patients more information, to help them more. It's a great program, a lot better than HMOs, which give you the bare minimum to get you by.

DR. PATON: *I thought insurance was supposed to give people "peace of mind."*

MT: Well, that's what insurance sells, but unfortunately it's really about selling the bare minimum in most markets. Especially with group employers, they're trying to offer their people peace of mind for the lowest price available.

HMOs are the lowest level of health insurance. There is nothing lower—besides no insurance. You have seen people denied care; I have personally seen it and I have heard about it, in some cases because they didn't have a condition pre-certified. They went to see a specialist because they were having a symptom of some kind, but didn't go through their primary care doctor. You have to follow a large amount of steps to be able to get to the end of the road with an HMO if you have a serious condition, as opposed to being able to go directly to the specialist, to a main servicer of your ailment—or what you've been led to believe is your ailment.

If there is a highly specialized specialist in your field and this specialist is not a member of your HMO, you will not be able to get that service. With PPOs, Medicare, the PFFSs, the supplements, you can go to them, they give you that option. But with HMOs you are so limited it's almost a dangerous coverage; it's the most basic and almost misleading.

TYPES OF INSURANCE

- Preferred provider options (PPOs) allow you to go to any provider on the plan's list and cover a wide variety of services Some cover "outside" providers but will charge you a larger copayment for them.
- HMOs cost the least but also give you the least options. With and HMO, you have a primary care physician who acts as a "gatekeeper," determining what is medically necessary for you and when you should see a specialist. An HMO has to permit certain treatment, but can also rule against your doctor for treatments it deems too expensive.
- Medicare private-fee-for-service (PFFS) plans provide the same benefits as original Medicare with additional benefits and lower copayments. They may limit what doctors you can see and how often.

DR. PATON: *So, if someone reading my book has an HMO, what would you say?*

MT: With PPOs, you have options. You can educate yourself, explore your options about which doctors to go to and even conference with them to find out more about them. Do you want a guy who knows Fords to work on your Ford or someone who works on Toyotas? If you take your car to a general mechanic, he might not know what's wrong in your specific situation. That's how the HMO works: If you have something seriously wrong with your back or leg, will your primary doctor necessarily have that kind of knowledge or information? Probably not, but he/she will refer you to someone he/she thinks will know about it or someone in his/her group or network of doctors.

DR. PATON: *I've found that sometimes people come see me, and let's say I think they need an MRI. With HMOs I can't order it because I'm not in their network. So I tell them to go to their primary care doctor to order it so that the HMO will pay for it.*

MT: Right. With PPOs, you don't need to do that. With HMOs, everything has to be done through one guy—and he's usually kept so busy that he usually doesn't even know who you are.

DR. PATON: *Although I accept patients with HMOs on a cash basis, I try to never become an in network HMO provider because they're just too limited. I'm on one HMO plan, but I refuse to get on others. I can send this one patient for any test I want, but if someone comes in with another HMO and I try to order a test, they need to go to their primary. And the primary is put off by the HMO, who tells him he's ordering too many tests…*

MT: It cuts into their profitability.

DR. PATON: *Right. And so I'll send them, knowing that they need an MRI, the primary care doctor will say it wasn't approved by the insurance, and that will force us to go through physical therapy treatment, even if that's not the preferred treatment or the correct response to the problem. So now, the patient quits chiropractic, they go to physical* *therapy, in some cases they don't get better, then they have to order the test…it's a mess.*

MT: With an HMO, you're the puppet. Someone else is pulling the strings. That's the way it is. You're not in power. With a PPO and a lot of these other types of plans, you at least have the option to learn about what could benefit you. While you're self-educating you can only help yourself. You don't know how good a doctor is by how they speak—they may take the time to explain things (although that's less and less likely given the constraints put on office visits), but you don't always understand. Like lawyers and legalese. Doctors speak, but the average person doesn't understand. You have to do your own research, on the Internet, etc., to try to improve your own understanding.

DR. PATON: *Why is it so much money for somebody to have individual insurance with a $500 deductible PPO? I had a BCBS PPO with a $500 deductible. They raised the price every single five-month period even though we only had one doctor visit in an entire year. Why?*

MT: Profitability. People who are self-insured, who have to get their own insurance, represent the group that is by far the insurance companies' largest profit margin. Because they know you have no other options, no group, no employer. They know you have to swallow the pill and pay the money. You are the reason that insurance companies make the most money. Some people like you don't use the coverage; you have it just so you can sleep better at night.

DR. PATON: *My recommendation to people—let me know if you agree—is to go with a high deductible with their insurance company and an MSA, the medical savings account, where it's tax deductible, so whatever you spend you can deduct from your taxes. Would you recommend that?*

MT: It all depends on your conditioning. A lot of people will do better with a high deductible plan with co-payments. Some with anticipated medical needs, the high-deductible health plan with a tax deductible medical savings account will benefit at least 50% of the U.S. just due to the sheer fact that it's pre-taxed money going in, and because it bears interest in most cases up to a standard 4%, so if you're not spending the money it's gaining money for you. Financially that's sound.

Secondly, if you want to spend money on your medical needs once you reach a certain point, it caps. You don't spend any more out of pocket whether it's for prescriptions or medical equipment, doctors, specialists, hospital visits. People who are planning families, people with two or more children, that will be a beneficial plan. But for a single person in the 20-year range, a few co-payments would be more beneficial. Again, for the majority of families, the high deductible health plan is a brilliant idea when combined with the MSA.

DR. PATON: *We were faced with one of those tough situations. My wife's COBRA insurance (from her previous job) was going to terminate in one year so we looked into adding her on our BCBS—the PPO (she originally had individual group insurance through her job). Since she had previous C-sections, they put a C-section rider on the insurance, which said they wouldn't pay for any C-sections. So we were going to have another baby and we knew the baby would need delivery by C-section, so we were going to have to pay for the whole in-patient surgery, hospital room and everything, all out of pocket. That's just wrong.*

I hear it in my office all the time from patients who change insurance and the new insurance has riders that deny coverage for an issue or complaint they had years ago.

MT: It's a sad state of affairs that Medicare insurance is so much better than traditional individual or group insurance. Insurance now can look at your information from years back and point out any "risks" they're not willing to accept. They tell you you'll have to deal with it yourself. That's the whole thing with insurance—if something doesn't meet their profitability they deny the claim. Anything they can deny, they will. It comes down to a business form. They'll add waivers, riders, clauses, anything they can to give you the least amount of coverage for the highest profitability when it comes to individual coverage. With group coverage, they can't do that.

DR. PATON: *Why?*

MT: Because they're not allowed to underwrite individuals. They underwrite the entire group when they accept the group.

DR. PATON: *So the individual is the true loser in all this.*

MT: Yeah, they can pick on you. You're the guy standing alone in the alley with the whole gang staring at you. Because the insurance company is just a gang of warriors—actuaries, managers, etc., told to maximize profits while still providing a slight peace of mind.

But God forbid you should have an accident, God forbid one of your children gets hurt… basic coverage won't be there when you need it the most. It might help cover the huge bills in some cases, but definitely not in all cases. Take underwriting, for example. There's a 28- to 32- page booklet in most cases, which doesn't even include the riders. That can get extremely complicated and it's so convoluted you really don't understand what you're getting. You really need an attorney *and* an insurance agent to explain it to you, because the insurance agent will not be focusing on the legalities involved (purposely or not).

The insurance companies put a layer of protection between the patient and the corporation. Part of the responsibility falls to the employer who is signing people up or signing the original contract for the group coverage. It becomes a little disturbing that they're not getting the coverage they think they've got. The employers think they're getting a good base coverage, but they take shortcuts on it. They know the shortcuts are saving people money and that the coverage may hurt one person out of the whole group and that's what happened to Moore [Note: referring to Michael Moore's movie *Sicko*], where if he didn't have this one surgery it would have killed him over a year or two. Eventually Moore stood in front of the corporation, raised a ruckus, and they caved. Bad publicity for an insurance company is horrible publicity. You can only have good publicity.

MT: Furthermore, a lot of time, instead of paying a doctor or an ex-doctor or a retired doctor, they'll hire nurse practitioners to redirect the patients to tell them they don't need the coverage or the treatment. Unfortunately, it kills some people. But remember, insurance companies are in business to maximize profitability. They're not there to help everyone. They're primarily there to help maybe the majority of the people.

DR. PATON: *What do you think about the elderly population? Do we take care of them?*

MT: Better than we take care of the young population. The elderly automatically get Medicare, which is a good, basic coverage; they get hospital and doctor coverage. And there are many PPOs, etc., available to purchase on top of their Medicare plans to help reduce their risks again. There are also supplements to help reduce their risks.

DR. PATON: *I've got a friend and a patient who works at one of the big stores in the area. He does security there. He tells me stories about seniors who come into the store where he works and try to steal bottles of Tylenol. He told me it just happened last weekend again and asked me what he was supposed to do. He didn't want to arrest this old man who couldn't afford anything but was obviously in pain… He said that he could get fired for it, but he took $20 out of his wallet and said, "Here, buy the pills." What an awesome gesture.*

But he sees it all the time, with people who, as he says, are denied health coverage, the same people who raised us, took care of us, fought in wars for us…and on whom we're now turning our backs.

MT: It is hard to see. And first of all, Medicare doesn't cover everything either. They have deductibles so there comes a point for some people where they don't have the money to pay the deductibles, and because of the mindset created in this country over the last 30-45 years—"take your pills, take your pills"—they can't afford their medication anymore.

I always try to explain to people: when you hit x amount of dollars your coverage stops; Their jaws drop open, because if they stop paying for 2-4 months they're going to have absolutely no prescription drugs at all and they'll have to pay 100% out of pocket. "I don't know if I'll be able to eat!" they say. I hear this on a daily basis for our seniors. It's appalling. But this is what happens when you start having the larger separation from the upper class; it makes the middle class suffer and pay more.

It is the government's design that has the flaw. They originally charged people for Medicare $3 in 1965, and they had three or four times the benefits that they have now. Next to nothing for deductibles, next to nothing for co-pays, they had vision coverage, they had dental coverage, they had hearing coverage. Now with Medicare they have no vision, no dental, no hearing, they have high deductibles, and have to pay 20%. And Medicare-approved amounts would be designated by nurse practitioners and doctors who have retired and who have been trained by the old school methods, trained to deny a claim, say it's not a Medicare-approved amount, it's not medically necessary. It may not be medically necessary in their eyes, but it may be medically important to that person.

DR. PATON: *You said you're a Part D specialist?*

MT: Yes. Part D is the prescription drug program on Medicare. I specialize in senior care; 20% of our clients run into this coverage gap and can't afford the medications. A lot of these seniors for the past three decades have had the idea that this is the insurance you have, take it or leave it, and when they join Medicare and have all these other options (like supplements, HMOs, PPOs), they don't know what to do because they're not educated on the terminology and insurance coverages. When you've been fed by someone else for thirty years and then all of a sudden they say, "Feed yourself," what do you do?

DR. PATON: *What goes through your mind when a person tells you over the phone that they can't put food on their table after their deductible?*

MT: I try to come up with ideas for them.

DR. PATON: *Does everybody have compassion the way you do?*

MT: No. We have quotas we have to meet, specific numbers we're accountable for. But the main thing about my job is that it's about guidance and trustworthiness. Because if they can't trust you and you can't guide them, you really can't help them.

DR. PATON: *Now is that the company's description…or yours?*

MT: That's the insurance "motto."

DR. PATON: *Are there cases, maybe in other companies, where you've heard about unsympathetic workers…who say, "Sorry, there's nothing we can do"?*

MT: Even I have to say that to some people sometimes. It gets depressing sometimes but you have to look forward to the next person you may be able to help, get them better coverage, save them some money, something to avoid paying these outrageous deductibles, to afford some type of basic coverage so they can sleep better at night. But you can't do it in every situation. You honestly can't.

The only thing I can suggest is that people need to do more research on their own insurance but even more on the people we vote into office. If you knew who was donating to the campaigns of your politicians you'd be discouraged, because it's these companies and politicians who are trying to create a larger gap between the wealthy, the middle class and the poor. It's only going to be by changing leadership, and in my opinion we've had some poor leadership…

The 2003 Medicare Modernization Act was one of the worst things to happen for the average person, the average Medicare recipient. It made big insurance companies huge and made small insurance companies billionaires. This was a big business move. Right now many of the pharmaceuticals are running into problems—the GlaxoSmithKlines, the Bergan Brunswicks, the McCessins, they aren't doing as well as they used to in the past because they're finding out that these private insurance companies that are lobbying for these politicians have more money to lobby than they do.

DR. PATON: *I've talked to several pharmacists who have said that this isn't the business they wanted to get into and that it's a break-even business now.*

MT: It's bound to fail because you're going to have people leaving that field. They're going to find out that they won't be able to make the same kind of money they did in the past (usually $75-100,000 a year, which is a decent wage) as a chemical compound specialist. And they know more than any primary or specialist I've ever met because that's their job. They know how the chemicals combine with each other and affect an average person.

DR. PATON: *Can you share any particularly difficult insurance-related experiences you've had, maybe experiences that would help our readers know what to watch out for?*

MT: This actually happened very recently with a PART D prescription coverage. The person had not enrolled in time, they were just diagnosed with cancer (9-07), and needed to get highly specialized medication. I notified this woman that by Medicare's rules (again, set in place by the U.S. government), I could not allow her to apply for coverage or she would be turned down for coverage until November 15th and that coverage would not go into effect until January 1. So that means she would have a four-month window where she would be receiving cancer treatments and paying for them out-of-pocket, probably spending everything she's ever worked for.

The one thing I've heard about recently that's helping people is taking out reverse mortgages to pay for medical bills...but having to reverse-mortgage your house, having to repay a mortgage in your elder age? But that's the only way some people are able to pay for their medications. This government program locks them out of getting prescription coverage. Otherwise they have to order them from Canada and the U.S. is trying to put embargoes on ordering drugs from Canada. They're trying to block them but they're unsuccessful at this point.

DR. PATON: *And why are they "locking" people out on these plans?*
MT: Again, it's a government program. Remember, insurance replaces fear. They put a lock on it to keep payments in check. And not only that, this woman would have to pay a penalty. They put a 1% penalty per month on the standard Medicare prescription drug cost to try and "steer" people into joining it in advance.

DR. PATON: *So you mean that even if you join Medicare you don't have access to the Part D...*

MT: You have to join Part D coverage when you join Medicare. Otherwise, if you postpone it until later, there is a lockout period, and they will only allow forty-five days per year for someone to come into the plan—and then they penalize them for joining late.

DR. PATON: *So, in this woman's case, if she waited the forty-five days...*

MT: I don't know. She left the phone crying because I told her I couldn't do it, that they would not approve her. I have to apply to Medicare for someone to get the coverage and if you don't fall under their guidelines, I can't help you.

DR. PATON: *So she was locked out...*

MT: I think so. Sometimes Medicare makes some judgment calls to assist people if you call them directly, but I don't know what happens there, once it's out of my hands. I had a gentleman from Florida who had an HMO plan. Great plan, but he wanted to visit a specialist and did not realize that without seeing his primary care physician he was going to be paying huge bills. He called me screaming, "I can't pay this $1,100 bill. I can't eat." And I literally could see him not being able to eat. He didn't go through the right channels, probably didn't know the right way to do things, or had an insurance agent who was too much in a hurry to explain things to him…but he did not get directed properly through his HMO channel and ended up with a huge bill.

On the theory behind insurance, I spoke to one insured who told me he's been healthy for thirty years, that he'd hadn't seen a doctor in ten years. He works on a farm, and had been paying insurance year after year. He called me to ask how supplements can charge hundreds of dollars if you're not using them. I tried to explain to him what "community rated" was, and the associated fees. I told him it's what the whole group in an area uses. So he notified me that he was going to go uninsured.

Prices have gone up, coverage has gone down. They keep forcing more and more people to make tough decisions—eat or pay coverage to buy pills. Back when Baby Boomers were making political statements, there was pot, then cocaine, then ecstasy, and now pharmaceuticals. They're not illegal but equally as dangerous. Drugs are more accessible, legalized, and available by prescription.

Most of the big insurance companies are trying to do things, developing programs, advancements in their own communities, advance consumerism, trying to spread the word on high deductible health plans with MSAs. Because it is a way to help people save money, and get healthcare. But people have to know about finances in the first place to take advantage of these programs. They need to do their own research instead of depending on other people to tell us what we need to know and to know for us.

Insurance: A solution

Let's say that a family pays $950 per month in healthcare for a PPO with a $500 deductible. That totals $11,400 per year in healthcare costs. The amount that would have been used is approximately $3,000 (at most) in an otherwise healthy individual. Remember, that's $3,000 if we didn't even have insurance and had to pay out of pocket! So, in essence, we have spent $8,400 too much in healthcare. Multiply that over twenty years and that number becomes $168,000. Then add on interest that the money would have generated—over $200,000! That's $200,000 that could have been used for retirement, our kids' education, a house, or—yes—preventative healthcare.

The bottom line is that we're paying way too much in insurance to have low deductibles or low co-pays when we should have high deductible insurance that costs significantly less. With any health insurance, the only health professional we should see in network is our medical doctor. This allows for expensive tests or surgeries to be covered. All other doctor visits should be paid in cash. These include the chiropractor, eye doctor, and dentist.

Let's say we switch to high deductible insurance, around $5,000. Rather than costing us $950 per month for a family it will now cost $180, a savings of $770 per month. The typical chiropractic case costs around $1,500 (for approximately 3 months) and then monthly charges (for maintenance) can cost anywhere from $50-$100. So the first year as a chiropractic patient may cost approximately $2,000 and each year after that approximately $800 per year.

Add on an eye doctor and dentist visit, and you may spend $3,000 per year in out-of-pocket healthcare costs. Don't forget, we saved approximately $770 per month by going with high deductible insurance, so our healthcare costs for the year have been offset by what we saved over just three short months. There are nine more months in the year, so that adds up to a lot of savings.

Perhaps the most important thing to remember is to have discipline and not spend that extra money. Ideally, one could set up a money market account and still pay the amount saved by using this plan into that account. So if our new insurance costs $180 per month, we're paying that to the insurance company AND we're putting the extra $770 into the money market (as if we still had an insurance payment of $950 per month).

By making that payment every single month, you will find yourself decidedly richer. At the end of the year, leave 20% in the account and use the rest for retirement accounts, college savings funds, or to take a nice vacation. After all, relaxation is sometimes the best treatment for high stress times!

CHAPTER FOUR

VACCINES: NOT THE LIFE-SAVERS WE WERE LED TO BELIEVE

What's the real story?

Most people have bought into the myth that without vaccination, a child will die, and that living without a vaccine is actually more dangerous than getting one. I disagree, and I'll tell you why.

First of all, let's look at how many new vaccines have been created in the last generation. Even the youngest teachers at our children's schools haven't received all the newest vaccines. Does that make them dangerous to their students? Does that make each of us a danger to our children because we haven't received these shots? I don't believe so, but if it were even the slightest bit reasonable, wouldn't we all be told to hurry to our doctors to get all the vaccines we missed but that our children have received?

The U.S. government is telling us that our children must be vaccinated to attend school in this country, and laws are being established as this book is being written to make sure that that happens. This is a significant miscarriage of justice, based on the fact that most people have been brainwashed into believing that it's dangerous *not* to be vaccinated. We're being swayed by fear to accept the drug company's version of what is good for us and our children. But the truth is that not only do vaccines *not* serve as lifetime immunity, they are actually dangerous to our health.

WHAT HAPPENS WHEN YOU SAY,
"NO, THANK YOU"?

A friend of ours just took her son to the pediatrician. When she indicated that she wasn't comfortable having her son vaccinated, the pediatrician shrugged and said, "People are dying of chicken pox. So, if you want your son to die…" Naturally our friend capitulated to pressure from a "trusted medical professional" even though it went against what she believed.

As I write this book, arguments over whether the soaring rates of autism and a host of other diseases could be caused by vaccines are in the news almost daily, showing no indication of stopping any time soon. Parent groups and allies accuse scientists and public health officials of hiding information to cover up mistakes, and scientists are offended—and in some cases intimidated—by an onslaught of e-mail, Internet slurs, and unprecedented criticism.

Virtually all medical professional societies, such as the Centers for Disease Control and Prevention, the World Health Organization, and the Institute of Medicine, have continued to state that there is no evidence vaccines cause autism. Yet, in the meantime, the rates of autism continue to rise, and since I expect the battle will rage for quite some time, the only thing we can do is take a stand for what we feel is right.

How to say "no"
On a personal level, my wife and I have been as confused and scared as any other parents out there. We were opposed to vaccines, but one in particular—the rotavirus vaccine. Rotavirus is a virus that causes diarrhea and most often infects infants and young children, and is particularly a problem for child-care centers and children's hospitals. Most children have had a rotavirus infection by the time they are five years old.

According to www.kidshealth.org, diarrhea brought on by rotavirus causes over half a million deaths every year around the world, especially in developing nations that lack sufficient healthcare and nutrition resources. They recommend frequent hand washing as the best tool to limit the spread of rotavirus infection, and quote the American Academy of Pediatrics (AAP), which suggest including RotaTeq, the rotavirus vaccine, in routine infant immunizations. It has been shown to prevent around 75% of infections and 98% of the illness' most severe cases.

Hoping to discuss the vaccine with our pediatrician, we arrived at her office for our scheduled visit to determine how our one-year-old child was progressing. We were unconvinced that vaccinating was the right thing to do, had a stack of research on hand, and were planning to talk to the pediatrician about our concerns.

When the nurse entered the room with several hypodermic needles filled with vaccines, we told her that we were not ready to take that step since our child was healthy and we were going to wait to think about it. She said "Okay," in a voice heavily laden with sarcasm, left the room and called for the pediatrician.

When the doctor entered, we brought out the stack of research we had amassed. We told her that the more we had thought about it, the more certain we were that we did not want to proceed with the rotavirus vaccine for our son, and were unsure about proceeding with any of the vaccines in the future.

As parents, my wife Janice and I try to do the best for our children, and part of that concern and love means trying to protect them from illness and harm. So when we brought our concerns to the pediatrician, we expected support for our efforts in grappling with this difficult issue. This was not at all what happened. The pediatrician was not pleased with our questions; she listened but then turned to us and said, *without hesitation*, "The vaccine has been proven safe." The pediatrician went on to tell us, as we stood gaping, that if we didn't vaccinate our son within one month, she would not see him anymore.

She was clearly put out and her tone was demanding and irritated as she went on to talk about the necessity and benefits of the hepatitis B vaccine. When we told her that we had elected not to get that vaccine either, she wanted an explanation. I argued, admittedly with some sarcasm myself, that I did not see the point since the only ways in which one can become infected with hepatitis (inflammation of the liver, caused by a virus or a toxin and characterized by jaundice, liver enlargement, and fever) are by having unprotected sex or by sharing intravenous drug needles. In an effort to lighten the mood,

I told her I wasn't planning on letting my one-year-old have sex anytime soon or share needles with any 2-year-old junkies.

There are many variations of hepatitis: A, B, C, D, E, F, G and H, but the current "necessary" form of the shot vaccinates only for Hepatitis B. So, even if the vaccination *did* prevent some hepatitis without potentially disastrous side effects, it would do nothing to prevent any of the other hepatitis infections.

Unfortunately, the doctor didn't find much humor—or logic—in my response and was actually quite offended. In an effort to understand her point of view, I asked, "Why would you vaccinate an infant who is not at a high-risk age for contracting this infection?" I could not have been more shocked by her answer. She responded by saying that the hepatitis vaccine required three separate doses, with a specified interim of time in between each dose. Since it was too difficult to get teenagers to come back for all three necessary doses, they vaccinate infants because it is easier to require it along with all the other vaccines and there would be more compliance.

I was dumbfounded that she would accept this explanation as viable—that vaccines should be given to infants simply because it was expeditious—and also that she would expect us to buy into it, too. We felt under attack, made out to be irresponsible, uncaring parents for having these concerns.

Sure enough, we finally caved under the pressure—to an extent. We did allow a couple of the other vaccines to be given to our son, but stood firm on the rotavirus vaccine. I am convinced that it was partly because I'm in the medical field that my wife and I felt strong enough to stand by our convictions. We did fire the pediatrician whose policy did not allow for parental decision-making and found another one who was more in tune with our needs and beliefs. Our child has never received any more vaccines since that day, nor has any of my other children. But how many parents would simply give way, sign the forms, and go about their business, feeling that the doctor must be right and that their own concerns had no merit?

How many of us *do what we're told* when we hear words such as, "It's been researched" because we simply don't know what else to do?

As amazing as it seems now, as I stated earlier, within just a few months after this "discussion" with the pediatrician, the rotavirus vaccine *was pulled off the market*! Many people who have heard this story asked me if I ever called the pediatrician to say, "I told you so"? The answer is no because I know that this doctor is the one who has to live with herself and the decisions she made, and because I hope she has learned to be less rigid in her approach. I would advise anyone researching these matters to check out: www.russellblaylockmd.com. Dr. Blaylock is a board-certified neurosurgeon, author, and lecturer who offers brilliant explanations of many medical issues in our country.

The terrifying reality is that scientists and doctors promote treatments that are often undeserving of their promotion. In this case, the company who developed the vaccine for rotavirus was not only taken to court, where they lost their case, but was forced to create that multi-billion dollar fund for parents of the many children left permanently disabled by the vaccine.

Can you imagine how it feels to the parents of those children, parents who only wanted to protect them from harm? Can you imagine how it feels to have listened to the "educated medical professionals" and trusted them to provide the information to make an informed decision?

I can't.

Because what could be worse than watching our children living with the effects of a "medical mistake," having to live with the guilt of not having questioned on behalf of our offspring's well-being? A parent or guardian has to be able to take a stand when a person in authority decides what's best for our child, just as we all need to take a stand when it comes to our own healthcare. That's not always easy when that person is a doctor telling you that it's your decision, but that, in effect, you'd be making a big mistake. That's why you have to do your research and be armed with knowledge and a support system (in the form of a supportive physician).

What is the result of our having stood firm despite pressure from medical professionals and "scientific research"? I've already mentioned our son's consistent good health, and how I believe it is based on many factors.

For example, it's common knowledge that most children in daycare spread germs to each other on a daily basis and often spread illness around just as easily. When Tyler was born, Janice and I both worked full-time. I had just graduated from chiropractic college and Janice taught school, so Tyler was, from the age of six months, exposed to germs not only during daycare, but also through my wife after a long day of teaching kindergartners.

But Tyler has been really sick only once in his entire life. He has *never* had an ear infection, nor has he ever had a sore throat. You're probably wondering how this is possible. Kids get sick regularly, right? Wrong. Kids should be healthier than any of us.

As early as infancy, we weaken their immune systems by injecting far too many vaccines into these tiny, delicate bodies. Even the preservative that goes into the vaccine is extremely harmful. These same vaccines send the baby's immune system into shock.

In the average life of a child, there's no way he or she could possibly be exposed to the many viruses and bacteria that exist in a vaccine and are injected ALL AT ONCE! These injections can cause the immune system to become overloaded to the point of permanent damage.

Vaccines and polio

The majority of us have been immunized from the time we were infants, in the '50s, '60s and '70s. I imagine I will offend some readers with this statement, but I believe some of the people involved in the mass polio vaccination are still patting themselves on the backs to this day, even though times have changed. We know more than we did then. We know the harm that can be done. We need to think of our children before profits.

On October 27, 2002, the *Atlanta Journal Constitution* reported that according to the Centers for Disease Control, an outbreak of polio in the Dominican Republic and Haiti had been caused by a mutation of oral vaccine's weakened virus that returned it to full strength. This is a clear indicator that we're all still at risk for developing polio, vaccinated or not, isn't it? After all, there is a mutated strain that was never included in the vaccine we received, floating around in the world right now.

In fact, it does not mean that, because it is not the vaccine that is the "cloak that protects us;" it is proper water treatment protocols.

Polio is actually a virus that lives and proliferates in the "gut" of the infected person, and can only be transferred from person to person through contact with infected fecal material. Polio lives in fecal material, and fecal material was flushed into the sewer. Years ago, when sewers backed up during a storm, drinking water became contaminated and was consequently consumed.

Today, drinking water—at least in this country—is treated (decontaminated for consumption) to a far greater extent than it was forty years ago. That's why polio has been all but eradicated in the U.S. But that's also why, until potable water is treated properly, we will never fully eradicate polio in third world countries.

There is also the fact that viruses mutate; that's what they do. As long as they continue to mutate, we will never be truly protected. Being vaccinated can never really protect us fully because newly-mutated forms of the virus are always manifesting. We cannot be vaccinated for mutating forms that have not yet manifested.

Theoretically, we're all at tremendous risk (as the drug companies would have us believe) because these viruses are "merely a plane ride away." So why aren't we experiencing a resurgence of polio in this country? Because this country's water treatment protocols all but completely remove us from that threat. And if someone traveling from a country such as the Dominican Republic were to carry a wild form of the mutated virus to the U.S., a form for which we are not vaccinated, the chances of coming in contact with the contaminated feces is so unlikely as to be almost impossible.

What I'm suggesting is not that polio—or any other virus—is not a potential, if highly unlikely, danger but that there are much safer ways of dealing with diseases than injecting dangerous chemicals into a child's body.

PRO-VACCINE SITES LIKE THESE KEEP OUR FEARS ALIVE

Polio.com asserts that the disease has been just about eradicated from the U.S. and the Western hemisphere thanks to vaccines. It also says that since polio is still active in other parts of the world, just one infected person could bring it into the U.S.and start another epidemic— *if* we weren't protected by vaccines.

When we hear or read statements like these, instead of reacting with fear, what we need to do is consider the source. In this case, it should come as no surprise that the other Website address for polio.com is www.vaccineplace.com.

Environmental links to vaccines

Links between vaccines and the environment are everywhere. Some sources say that the mercury in vaccines has no link to any health problems in children. Though it has nothing to do with vaccines, that's what they said about lead, fifty years ago. Lead is similar to mercury in that although mercury is a transition metal, it is a heavy metal with the same affinity to neurological tissue in the brain as lead does.

Before I became a chiropractor, I worked as an environmental chemist for one of the most well known environmental companies in the U.S. I had just been accepted into the University of South Florida College of Public Health, and was majoring in environmental chemistry. One of my jobs was to assist the project manager in writing technical reports to our clients, such as the FDOT (Florida Department of Transportation), describing how the site clean-ups were progressing. Most of the time I was on the road, going to different environmental remediation (clean-up) sites, where I would take soil and water samples and analyze them in a mobile laboratory with the use of a gas chromatograph. The samples came from huge pits dug by heavy machinery, and I would let the machinery operators know if they needed to dig farther or when they finally hit a clean area.

Occasionally, to get a break from being in the lab and observe the progress, I walked out to the pit. On some job sites, I, along with the entire crew, had to be in full Tyvek and use a respirator. Tyvek is a brand of flashspun high-density polyethylene fibers, a synthetic material, which is a registered trademark of the DuPont Company. They are those white one-piece outfits that cover your entire body and have hoods—when you wear one, you look like you're in a nuclear fallout area. I remember one job site where several hundred 55-gallon drums of lead-based paint had been buried in the ground and were consequently being excavated.

Let's look at what happens to the brain so we can understand the impact that heavy metals like lead can have.

A study on lead poisoning and brain cell function in *Environmental Health Perspectives* ("Lead Poisoning And Brain Cell Function," Goldstein GW, 1990, 89, 91-94) states that there are two parts of the brain, broadly divided into neurons and endothelial cells, tissues composed of a single layer of smooth, thin cells that line the heart, blood vessels, lymphatics, and serous cavities.

According to the author, lead can accumulate in the brain, and high-level exposure to the metal can lead to a loss of "normal barrier function." He states that a person's brain function can be negatively affected if exposed to large amounts of lead when he or she is a toddler. He goes on to note that lead is often ingested at a young age, when the brain's synaptic connections are changing significantly, and such lead poisoning can disrupt the development of neural networks with no outward symptoms.

Lead is considered a heavy metal, and heavy metals, when absorbed through the skin or drank through contaminated water, migrate through the body and become absorbed by what's called our white matter. The central nervous system is made of three solid components: white, gray and *substantia nigra*. White matter is the tissue through which messages pass between different areas of gray matter within the central nervous system.

To use a computer network analogy, if the gray matter is an actual computer itself, the white matter is represented by the network cables that connect the computers together. The nerve fibers of white matter are surrounded by a substance that helps messages pass quickly from place to place. This is also the material that makes up the brain and spinal cord.

Gray matter, which has no myelin, is the material that makes up the nerves that course throughout your entire body. Nerves that consist of gray matter can be severed and regenerate. White matter *cannot* regenerate. So, once a heavy metal becomes absorbed by the central nervous system or white matter, major neurological damage has been done. What constitutes "major neurological damage"? Problems and diseases such as autism, Parkinson's, Alzheimer's, and many more.

Looking back to the 1950s, when the Florida Department of Transportation painted new lines on all the roads with lead-based paint, we can see that repercussions would someday manifest. Indeed, when FDOT finished painting all the lines, they simply buried all the unused, lead-based paint. At that time, they didn't know (or didn't care, or didn't care to find out) that burying high concentrations of lead-based paint would have dire consequences to the environment and/or to humans. They just did it.

Oh, I imagine someone might have made an attempt to keep it from happening or to indicate that there would be negative environmental effects. But behind every organization there is a system that launches the line we hear so often: "There's no scientific evidence that would suggest..." In this case, that meant abject denial of the possible consequences.

So all that lead-based paint ended up in the ground. It is no surprise that now, fifty years later, those buried drums have completely rusted through and the paint is not only leaching (being absorbed) into the environment, but is also leaching directly into the water table.

At one particular job site, we not only found severe lead contamination in the ground, but we identified it in the drinking water in the vicinity of the contamination. Whether it was above or below the legal limits, there was *lead* in the water. The local people were drinking lead-contaminated water, the same lead that is known to cause neurological damage in human beings. Why? Because the government made a decision fifty years ago based on insufficient evidence.

And who pays the price? We do.

According to a study in the *New England Journal of Medicine* (*Environmental Lead Exposure: A public health problem of global dimensions*, Shilu Tong; Yasmin E. von Schirnding; Tippawan Prapamontol, 322, pp. 83-88, Jan 11, 1990), exposure to lead has been a "serious problem" in developing countries. Awareness of the problem has been growing, but few regulations have been put in place to counter the problem. The study goes on to note that higher lead levels in childhood were "significantly associated" with, among other traits, absenteeism, lower language test scores and poorer hand-eye coordination in high school students.

So, to return to the link between vaccines and the environment, I find it curious that we would consider using substances in vaccines that could be harmful to our children based on only "what might be true" or has "not been proven" yet.

On what facts is the law requiring all children to be vaccinated based? Is it negligence or denial or sheer stupidity that allows us to believe in the same government that "didn't know enough" about lead in the fifties telling us now that vaccines are "proven safe"? Isn't it entirely possible that these vaccines are more harmful than helpful, based on all the studies done in the last few decades?

Think about it: 50 years ago the government told people that it was acceptable to bury lead-based paint in the ground. Most people trusted the government, but they should have asked more questions. How many people have drank water for years that contained lead? And how many people currently have residual side effects from the lead contamination? We may never know. The point is that the government isn't always right, and ultimately YOU are responsible for your and your family's health and well-being.

But we are in a bind because even though vaccines have been found to utilize a component known to cause permanent neurological damage in growing children, we are being told to vaccinate our children. And we are still injecting our children with substances potentially so dangerous that we have to suit up on job sites to avoid contamination by them.

Does that make sense?

Vaccines and mercury

Mercury is another case in point. Compare it to lead by looking at a periodic table (find "lead," move two spots to the left and you'll see "mercury"). Mercury is a heavy metal so toxic that job sites in where mercury contamination is in evidence require wearing full Tyvek, respirators, and several layers of gloves—just as lead does. We've known about this extreme hazard *for years*, but for years we've injected our children with vaccines containing mercury.

So, I ask again, how does that make any sense to anyone?

On their Website, www.chop.edu, the Children's Hospital of Philadelphia Vaccination Center refutes the claim that mercury in vaccines can be harmful because it is *ethyl*mercury, not *methyl*mercury, which can be toxic to humans in high doses. They claim that ethylmercury, the type of mercury used in the influenza vaccine, can be broken down and excreted much more quickly, and is therefore "unlikely" to accumulate and damage the body.

But, as is the case with so many drugs, we do not always know the true effects of substances in the body until years later, when the damage has already been done. Since mercury has an increased preference for neurological cells, it will be found in neurological tissues such as the brain, *not in the blood*, so the blood testing done in studies is not a reliable method of detecting levels of toxicity.

Mercury is also known to do permanent neurological damage to the central nervous system. If you were born before 1970, you'll probably remember those mercury-filled thermometers. When they broke, the first thing the school nurse or your parent would yell is, "Stay away! Don't touch that stuff!" It could be absorbed through your skin.

We knew way back then that mercury was dangerous but continued to inject it into our children, and we still use it to fill cavities in our teeth even though the mouth is one of the primary places through which we absorb bacteria, etc. (For information on this subject, read *Tooth Truth…If You Want To Be Healthy Don't METAL With Your Teeth*, by Frank J. Jerome, D.D.S., New Century Press; August 15, 2000. It has groundbreaking research that looks into the risks of using mercury and other metals in fillings and the degenerative diseases that can result.)

The National Vaccine Information Center's Website, www.909Shot.com, notes that in 1982, the FDA called for thimerosal, the form of mercury used in vaccines since the '30s, to be removed from over-the-counter products because of its toxicity. In 1999, the FDA found that exposure to mercury from vaccines surpassed the EPA's safety guidelines. It seemed that the government hadn't been fully analyzing the amount of mercury in the new vaccines they'd been adding to the mandatory childhood schedule, and failed to recognize how much mercury a child would be exposed to over the course of a full vaccination regimen.

In 1999, due to pressure from the FDA, many companies did indeed begin to remove thimerosal from their products, but some products that indicate they are "thimerosal-free" still contain trace amounts, and thimerosal continues to be used in some vaccines.

Though some neuro-developmental disorders such as autism have similar symptoms as mercury poisoning, and though it is well established that mercury is a neurotoxin harmful to babies *in utero* and to the developing brains of children, and though there is a public health advisory from the government about the risks of eating mercury-containing seafood, there continues to be no public health advisory about the risks of exposure to mercury in vaccines.

Vaccines and animals: What else can we learn?

Deirdre Imus, founder of The Deirdre Imus Foundation For Pediatric Oncology, advocate for the environment and children's health, has set the stage for taking on challenging issues. Articles on her website (www.dienviro.com) are a wealth of information on many subjects, including that of vaccination and its possible relationship to the rising levels of autism in our youth.

I was shocked to learn from one of Imus' articles that the mercury-containing preservative we've been discussing above— thimerosal—which had been used in animal vaccines for over fifty years, *was removed from all animal vaccines way back in 1992.* Imus states, "Studies have provided evidence that the over-vaccination of dogs and cats can result in numerous maladies including cancer, skin and ear conditions, arthritis, allergies, diabetes, aggression, behavior problems and other immune system dysfunctions…"

It is yet another case of injustice against our children that this substance not only remained in children's vaccines for another decade, but continues to remain in many vaccines today, such as influenza (at a level of 25 micrograms) and tetanus shots (at a level of 25 micrograms).

At any level, it's too much.

The scientific community has known for years that thimerosal is a proven carcinogen. One study (Kravchenko, AT, et al, *Zh Mikrobiol Epidemiol Immunobiol*, 1983 (3):87-92) even concluded that it was able to change the properties of cells.

As Imus states, vaccines contain 50,000 ppb mercury, or 250 times more than substances that are considered hazardous waste. Even a "trace amount" in a vaccines could range from 600 to 2000 ppb.

Although the Centers For Disease Control and The Institute for Vaccine Safety both claim there are "no biological effects" from trace amounts (.3 micrograms) of mercury, Imus and others (including myself) question why we are not seeing any evidence-based ("conflict-free") studies to actually prove the safety of these "trace" amounts. In March 2005, Imus declared that he had questions about the *NEJM* study, which asserted that "over-vaccinating" posed no health concerns for the general public.

This is yet another case in which one of the very organizations that originally insisted a product was safe changed its tune down the line—when it was too late for millions of children and adults. Though the American Academy of Pediatrics had stated that according to well-documented studies, mercury in vaccines did not in any way cause autism or other neurological disorders, it has now become one of the filers of the lawsuit against the EPA. Too many parents are unaware of these facts, bringing their children to pediatricians and trusting in their recommendations for vaccinations as "safe" procedures.

I'm the first to admit it's hard to know what to do. Reading articles in respected journals and magazines should be educational, but there is no guarantee that the information is *good* information. For example, a friend recently told me about an article in *Momsense*, published by MOPS (Mothers of Preschoolers). It appeared in a section called "Health Matters." The pediatrician who wrote the article was answering the following question: "I'm concerned because I heard that vaccines can cause autism and other serious problems. Some of my friends chose not to immunize their babies. Do I need to vaccinate my baby?"

Although the article made an attempt to educate without

making recommendations, my friend was confused by its basic message to the parent, that "it's your call" whether to get vaccines or not. The distressing aspect of this advice is that the physician made statements in direct opposition of each other, confusing parents trying to "make the right call." The writer stated that medical studies have shown no link between autism and mercury exposure. In another statement, she countered the first one by recommending that the reader ask for a thimerosal-free vaccine from her child's doctor.

In the short space of one article, this respected medical doctor had encouraged parents to make their own decisions; said there was no link between autism and thimerosal; and specifically suggested that parents request vaccines without thimerosal.

Is it any wonder that in the attempt to educate ourselves, we find ourselves more bewildered than ever?

Diseases of the brain and heavy metal poisoning

In an article on Alzheimer's disease in the peer-reviewed scientific journal *Neuroendocrinology Letters* (J. Mutter, J. Naumann, C. Sadaghiani, R. Schneider, *Alzheimer's Disease: Mercury As Pathogenetic Factor And Apolipoprotein E As A Moderator,* 25, 5; 331-339, Oct. 2004), the authors note studies that showed deceased Alzheimer's patients with higher levels mercury in their brains, and living patients with the same in their blood. They also note experimental studies that found that trace amounts of mercury could cause nerve cell changes that are characteristic of Alzheimer's—though other metals, even in low concentrations, could not.

Additionally, the authors state that cumulative exposure to mercury could lead to cognitive impairment years later. In layman's terms, this means that ingestion of mercury can take years to have an effect on our bodies—in fact, up to 30-50 years before symptoms of mercury poison manifest.

Vaccines, mercury and the law

We now know that Americans are regularly exposed to unsafe levels of mercury from environmental sources, including power plant emissions and by eating contaminated fish, and EPA investigators have estimated that over 600,000 newborns are born each year over-exposed to unhealthy mercury levels *in utero*.

We also know that the EPA not only ignored the advice of its own Children's Health Public Advisory Committee and nearly 700,000 overwhelmingly negative public comments, but also chose to overlook the annual economic costs that methyl mercury toxicity incurs through lost productivity due to physical and mental impairment.

What will happen when this significant loss of intelligence continues throughout the lifetime of exposed children? Will our economic competitiveness and productivity decrease as more of the population requires extra time, attention and special education? And what do we think will happen when infants whose brains are still rapidly developing are exposed to vaccines with "trace"—but still unsafe—amounts of mercury?

What stands out are the items about how the same groups who made a case *for* a vaccine or drug often, in a total about-face, denounce it at a later date. Don't get me wrong—I'm encouraged by their candor and honesty to state the facts as they eventually see them. But my concerns are still as real as ever: How can we possibly know what to believe, and why does it take so long for these organizations to come forward?

This goes to show that we cannot base personal health decisions on one study or on one medical professional's point of view.

Importantly, the American Association for Health Freedom (AAHF, at www.healthfreedom.net) is starting a new initiative, The Coalition Against Mandatory Vaccination, led by Dr. Sherri Tenpenny, AAHF President and well-known authority on vaccines. This initiative will partner with state chapters to ensure that philosophical exemptions to vaccines are enacted (and protected) in all states. Currently all states and the District of Columbia offer a medical exemption, all but two states offer a religious exemption (MI, WV), and only eighteen states offer a philosophical exemption. Dr. Tenpenny says she has been receiving hundreds of stories (such as the previous one) about out-of-control and bullying physicians who insist on their patients being vaccinated.

As unbelievable as it sounds, attacks on religious, philosophical and personal exemptions to vaccinations in America are increasing, along with attempts to *force* vaccination. They are being led by vaccine patent-holders like Paul Offit, M.D., and others who are creating an organization called People for Immunization, supposedly the source for "real information" about vaccines. Dr. Tenpenny, head of the Coalition Against Mandatory Vaccination, has said that she believes that People for Immunization's "hidden agenda" aims to eliminate vaccine exemptions an force vaccinations onto home-schooled children.

Dr. Tenpenny also notes that mandatory vaccination increases the cost of healthcare for everyone, making it less attainable for all who need it, and that almost 32% of the CDC's annual budget ($2.1 billion in 2007) goes toward vaccines. She asserts that state-enforced vaccinations are intrusive, and that we should each have the right to decide what to do with our own bodies.

AAHF is working to establish state chapters in all 50 states. Its important mission is to secure "the right of the consumer to choose and the practitioner to practice." If you are a concerned parent or citizen who wants to fight obligatory vaccination, I urge you to go to www.healthfreedom.net, the Website of the American Association For Health Freedom.

Vaccines and Big Pharma

Drug companies contribute to the dilemma. They can be purposefully vague (some might even say "obstructive"), making it difficult for us to make the choices we need to make.

As an illustration, the following story has been reprinted in totality with the author's permission:

A MOTHER'S STORY

My name is Lyn Redwood. I reside in Atlanta, Georgia with my husband Tommy and three children, Hanna, Drew and Will. My husband and I are both health care professionals. My husband is a Physician and I'm a Nurse Practitioner. I also hold a Masters Degree in Community Health Nursing and I'm a member of our County's Board of Health and local Planning Commission.

My son, Will, weighed in at close to 9 lbs at birth.

He was a happy baby who ate and slept well, smiled, cooed, walked and talked, all by one year. Shortly after his first birthday he experienced multiple infections, lost speech, eye contact, developed a very limited diet and suffered intermittent bouts of diarrhea. He underwent multiple evaluations and was initially diagnosed with a global receptive and expressive speech delay and later with Pervasive Developmental Disorder, a form of autism.

I would have never made a correlation between my son's disability and vaccines until July 1999 when I read that a preservative, thimerosal, utilized in some infant vaccines, actually contained 49.6% mercury. The report went on to say that the FDA had determined that "infants who received thimerosal-containing vaccines at several visits may be exposed to more mercury than recommended by Federal Guidelines for total mercury exposure." As health care providers my husband and I constantly receive notices that adverse events have been reported with a drug or a product safety sheet has been revised. Why were no such notices sent out informing us that thimerosal preserved vaccines were exceeding federal guidelines for mercury exposure in infants?

It was in light of this information that I reviewed my son's vaccine record and my worst fears were confirmed. All of his early vaccines had contained thimerosal. From my research on mercury I have found it to be a potent human toxicant, which is especially damaging to the rapidly developing fetal and infant brain. While acceptable levels for exposure are published by Federal Agencies, mercury is a poison at any level.

The dose thought to be safely allowed on a daily basis by EPA is 0.1mcg per kilogram of body weight per day. At 2 months of age my son had received 62.5 mcg of mercury from 3 infant vaccines. According to EPA criteria, his allowable dose was only 0.5mcg based on his weight. He had received 125 times his allowable exposure on that one day. These large injected bolus exposures continued at 4, 6, 12 and 18 months to a total mercury exposure of 237.5 mcg. I also discovered that the injections I received during the first and third trimesters of my pregnancy and hours after the delivery of my son to prevent RH blood incompatibility also contained mercury.

(Lyn Redwood is the Co-founder and President of SafeMinds. Excerpted with permission from her testimony at the Government Reform Committee, July 18, 2000. Please see www.safeminds.org or read Evidence of Harm by David Kirby for more information.)

Like Lyn Redwood, I am a parent. And, as a parent, I can't help wondering what the causes of the majority of diseases in the world are. Granted, some are genetic and are predictable. But what about all of the autoimmune conditions out there, such as rheumatoid arthritis, asthma, scleroderma, lupus, etc.? Let's take a closer look at these.

The word "autoimmune" combines "auto," meaning "self, same or spontaneous," and "immune," resulting in the meaning "of, or pertaining to, the immune response of an organism against any of its own tissues, cells, or cell components." There are no medical or scientific explanations as to why we suffer from conditions such as asthma, lupus or rheumatoid arthritis. And that's where my brain says, "Wait a second…"

Technology has allowed us to put people on the moon, and aim a satellite traveling at 6 miles per second at a moving comet, which, with pinpoint accuracy, it successfully impacts. Yet we can't explain what causes autoimmune conditions?

All the medical field can say is that the culprit is a "dysfunctional immune system." Why would our immune system fight itself? Why would it destroy its own tissues, cells or cell components in some kind of automatic response if it were healthy, well exercised and adept at searching out and destroying cells which don't belong? If medicine can't give me a plausible cause for autoimmune conditions, I, as a responsible parent, must examine what we do to our immune system throughout our lives that may engender these conditions.

As parents of sick kids, we must ask the question, "Why did my child get asthma, autism, allergies, etc. when no one in our family's history ever had these?" Ask yourself, "What did we put into our child's body that could have caused such an illness?" Then list what you did give your child—from antibiotics to vaccines to the foods you fed the child.

If you're reading this and thinking how to play devil's advocate, you'd say, "Well, I got vaccines and nothing happened to me!" Then you'd need to ask yourself this: "Why do some children get fevers when they get vaccinated whereas others don't? Why do some children develop redness around the injection site when others don't? Why do some children vomit or go into seizures after receiving vaccines when others don't?"

The answer is that everyone's genetics are so vastly different that each person reacts differently to the chemicals injected into his/her body. That's where the danger comes into play. Redness, fever and vomiting are merely the symptoms we see on the outside. If the reaction is that profound, then what's happening on the inside that doesn't immediately present symptoms we can see?

The obvious place to look is the injection of vaccines into our bodies. If you've ever seen a person who suffers with rheumatoid arthritis or other autoimmune conditions, you know how horrible these diseases can be. And until I have a valid, reasonable explanation for autism and autoimmune conditions, I will not allow anyone to inject anything into my child, unless the situation is life-threatening.

CHAPTER FIVE

HOW ANTIBIOTICS AFFECT OUR HEALTH

Where do antibiotics come from and what are they for?
Antibiotics are actually natural substances released by bacteria and fungi into the environment, as a means of inhibiting other organisms—basically a process we could call chemical warfare on a microscopic scale.

Louis Pasteur (born in France in 1822) first discovered that most infectious diseases are caused by germs. Known as the "germ theory of disease," it is considered by many in the profession to be one of the most important discoveries in medical history. (As a chiropractor, although I have an appreciation for this discovery, I don't necessarily agree with the germ theory of disease, but I will discuss how it dramatically molded the way our medical system has evolved over the years.) Pasteur's work became the foundation for the science of microbiology, and included the observation that bacteria could be used to kill other bacteria.

In 1928, Sir Alexander Fleming, a Scottish bacteriologist, left a petri dish of Staphylococcus aureus uncovered while he went away on vacation and returned to find that mold had formed. He observed that colonies of the bacterium *staphylococcus aureus* could be destroyed by the mold *penicillium notatum*, proving that there was an antibacterial agent at work. This principle later led to medicines that could kill certain types of disease-causing bacteria inside the body. Penicillin is one of the earliest discovered and widely used antibiotic agents, derived from the penicillium mold.

The use of penicillin did not begin until the 1940s when Drs. Howard Florey and Ernst Chain isolated the active ingredient and developed a powdery form of the substance. Unlike previous treatments for infections, which often consisted of administering chemical compounds with high toxicity, such as strychnine and arsenic, antibiotics from microbes were found to have no or few side effects and high efficacy.

Four years after drug companies began mass-producing penicillin in 1943, microbes began appearing that could resist it. The first bug to battle penicillin was Staphylococcus aureus. Though often a harmless passenger in the human body, "Staph" aureus can cause illness, such as pneumonia or toxic shock syndrome, when it overgrows or produces a toxin.

It is probably safe to say that penicillin was originally seen as something of a panacea— that is, until the resistors showed up to squelch its potential. Today, one of the biggest problems related to antibiotics is that people don't understand how they work, when they work, and why they're using them. I believe we still suffer from that mentality which existed when penicillin first came on the market, the one that implies that antibiotics cure everything.

This false belief has led to the gross overuse of antibiotics, even though their use is not appropriate in most situations or for most types of symptoms. The fact is that only very specific antibiotics are fit for the jobs we assign them to do, because only very specific antibiotics are appropriate for killing specific types of bacteria.

The term "antibiotic" originally referred to any agent that could perform a biological activity against living organisms; however, "antibiotic" now refers to substances with anti-bacterial, anti-fungal, or anti-parasitical activity. But, again, most anti-bacterial antibiotics do not have any effect against viruses, fungi, or other microbes. Some are narrow-spectrum antibiotics, which means there is a narrow target they affect; some are more broad-spectrum and affect a wider range of bacteria.

As you probably know, there are many antibiotics available to us: oral antibiotics (which are simply ingested), intravenous antibiotics (used in more serious or systemic cases), or topical antibiotics (for example, in the form of eye drops or ointments). The effectiveness of individual antibiotics varies with the location of the infection, the ability of the antibiotic to reach the site of infection, and the ability of the microbe to inactivate or excrete the antibiotic. Some antibacterial antibiotics destroy bacteria, whereas others prevent bacteria from multiplying.

Unfortunately, we seem to have forgotten the powerful truth that specific antibiotics perform specific functions. Even though science knows viruses are not affected by the use of antibiotics, they are often prescribed "just in case." And even though we know colds are generally virus-based, we want antibiotics to cure them. We've gotten to the point where we want antibiotics to cure anything and everything that's even slightly out of whack.

There are many reasons this isn't such a good idea. First, this overuse is creating antibiotic-resistant "super bugs" (like staph aureus, mentioned above), illnesses that do not respond to the use of antibiotics anymore. Secondly, our immune systems are weakened by our habitually throwing antibiotics at them instead of allowing them to do the work they're supposed to do to keep us healthy. Taking a course of antibiotics "just in case" does more damage—much more damage—to our systems than good.

How antibiotics suppress the immune system

In the right situations, antibiotics can be the correct course to follow. The key is to understand when the situation is right—or not—and not to prescribe antibiotics when the body's symptoms are telling us otherwise. The other critical element often missing when antibiotics are prescribed is that, much of the time, we can avoid needing antibiotics altogether if we keep our immune systems healthy and strong.

Our immune systems need to be exercised just like our cardiovascular systems do. If we've been sitting on the couch for six months, we can't expect to go out and run a marathon; the first time we try, we're going to hurt for a few days. The next time we go out and run, it will hurt again; we may feel exhausted, as if we're going to have a heart attack while we're running. Yet we make it through the run, expecting it to be difficult because we haven't exercised for so long. After several more uncomfortable "training runs," we feel a difference; it starts to get easier, more enjoyable. We get closer and closer to being in marathon shape.

Our immune systems are the same way; they need to be trained, exercised, and given the time to do what they are made to do. Antibiotics can seem like a quick fix, but ultimately it's like taking pills for weight loss—you might appear to be in shape but unless you eat right and exercise, the weight will come right back.

In a world of major antibiotic resistance, we all need to have immune systems that are in tiptop shape. If our immune systems do need help from time to time, there are often simple natural approaches and remedies that do the job successfully. The use of antibiotics remains a last resort.

Antibiotic mythology

There are several prevailing myths about the use of antibiotics:

> **Myth #1:** It is widely believed that antibiotics are responsible for the decline in infectious diseases. But according to the doctors who wrote *Beyond Antibiotics: 50 (or so) Ways to Boost Immunity and Avoid Antibiotics* (Keith Sehner, M.D., Lendon Smith, M.D., and Michael Schmidt, North Atlantic Books; 2nd Edition, 1994), this is not the case.
>
> The authors tracked the incidence of major infectious diseases from 1900 to 1973 (including measles, scarlet fever, tuberculosis, typhoid fever, pneumonia, influenza, whooping cough, diphtheria and polio) and found they were all in decline for several decades before the introduction of antibiotics or vaccines! In actuality, improved nutrition, sanitation and hygiene were far more important than "wonder drugs" or vaccines in reducing these diseases.
>
> **Myth #2:** Antibiotics are useful against colds and flu. By now most of us have heard that antibiotics

are only helpful for bacterial infections. But many physicians continue to prescribe them for viral conditions such as colds and flu, in an effort to "prevent secondary bacterial infection." Given the dangers of antibiotics, this may only worsen the situation and prolong recovery.

Myth #3: Antibiotics are harmless. Actually, nothing could be further from the truth. Not only does this misconception lead to over-prescribing, but the adverse effects of these medications often go overlooked. (Just check the *Physicians' Desk Reference*, the yearly reference guide that describes all current drug information.)

Other problems with antibiotics

The list of problems related to antibiotic usage is longer than you might think. Some are quite well known; others are not. I will not detail the entire list here, but will outline a few of the most adverse effects:

1. One of the most common side effects of antibiotics is allergic reaction, from hives to diarrhea—and even death. Not only can the drug cause reactions from mild to severe, but antibiotics contain sugar, additives, and chemical colors, which can also trigger reactions in some people.

2. Wide-spectrum antibiotics (those used to treat multiple conditions) are notorious for killing "good bugs" right along with the bad ones, the same way pesticides do. Some of these "good bugs" in our intestines help digest food, produce vitamins and maintain a balance of organisms that actually prevent harmful bacteria and yeasts from multiplying. Antibiotics will often prevent this balanced state. Parasitic infection, vitamin deficiencies, inflammation, malabsorbtion, food allergies…these

can all be due to defects in intestinal function brought about by antibiotic use.

3. There is also a backlash against widespread antibiotics use, which exists in the form of the development of resistant bugs. An article in *Science* magazine (August 1992) stated that hospitals around the world were "losing the battle" against drug-resistant infections such as staph, pneumonia, strep, tuberculosis and dysentery.

    How does this happen? Simply put, bacteria have the ability to mutate. Although antibiotics kill certain susceptible bacteria, the field is left open for mutant strains to multiply. It is a case of survival of the fittest, in which the use of antibiotics actually encourages the development of the mutant, drug-resistant "super bacteria."

4. For me, the most critical ability of an antibiotic is that it can suppress the immune system. This may sound paradoxical because we all know that the main purpose of antibiotics is to help the immune system. But there is clear evidence that people treated with antibiotics have more repeat infections than those who are not.

    Take, for example, children with multiple ear infections who are often treated over and over with different antibiotics until the physician "finds one that works." This ultimately inhibits the immune system's ability to fight the very conditions for which the antibiotics are being prescribed.

Parents of the kinds of children described above often come to my office desperate for some way to get off the antibiotic treadmill. I explain to them that, while it is true antibiotics act by inhibiting certain enzymatic processes of bacteria and by changing mineral balances, normal cells are also affected at the same time. When other conditions occur due to antibiotic usage, the overall effect is of a compromised immune system. (There is even recent speculation that since AIDS is a disease of an impaired immune system, repeated antibiotic use may be one of its causes. We'll have to see how that theory develops.)

There is one particular analogy I like to describe what can happen when course after course of antibiotics has been prescribed, but symptoms continue to persist:

A child goes to the doctor with repeated coughs and colds. Courses of antibiotics have not helped alleviate the symptoms. The doctor recommends that the child's tonsils and adenoids be removed. Voila! A few days later, the child is eating ice cream in the hospital with parts of his anatomy removed. Even now I hear doctors say that tonsils are not necessary and their removal will not have any future effects whatsoever.

Now, let's examine this situation using an analogy to a car traveling down the interstate:

You're driving down the interstate at 80 mph and your temperature gauge begins to rise because of a slow leak due to a loose hose clamp. You take the exit ramp and stop at the first auto parts store, where you pick up a can of Stop Leak and add it to the radiator. You're not sure where the leak is, but you figure what harm can it do, hoping that the Stop Leak will at least alleviate the symptom.

One month later, the slow leak starts again. You figure because it worked for a while the first time, you'll do the same thing, and you pour in another can of Stop Leak. This happens again two months later then five months later, and you continue to use the same protocol.

Finally, the fifth time, you're barreling down the highway when the temperature gauge goes way up. You're frustrated from dealing with this problem and you think, "This Stop Leak stuff isn't working. This time, I'm going to remove the wires connected to the temperature gauge so it never overheats again." In fact, you may just decide to sell your car altogether so you don't have to put up with this type of thing again.

Back to our sore throats... Does it really make sense to treat a symptom over and over *and over* with the same protocol that clearly doesn't work? Does it also make sense to say, "Well, this didn't work, so let's just remove the affected part altogether"? What would happen to a car without a hose clamp? Or without a temperature gauge to show us something's wrong? And what happens to a child without tonsils and adenoids?

For many years, parents were told that tonsils and adenoids were, for all intents and purposes, irrelevant. While the number of tonsillectomies and adenoidecotomies in the United States has decreased over the last 30 years, they are still the most commonly performed operation on children in our country, with over *400,000 per year*. Prior to World War II, removal of the tonsils was an American ritual and many children had this procedure performed as a matter of course or after one sore throat.

In my eyes, this is a travesty. Not only shouldn't we be risking 400,000 potentially unnecessary operations on children each year, but the medical community also shouldn't allow us to accept a lie. Medical professionals know just how important the tonsils and adenoids are in keeping the body healthy—yet many prefer we be kept in the dark.

According to www.kidsgrowth.com, tonsils and adenoids can actually fight infection by forming a tissue layer at the back of the throat, making them the "first line of defense" against germs trying to enter the body. The tonsils and adenoids are the main producers of virus- and bacteria-fighting cells and proteins before a child turns four.

This is another case of putting the needs of the medical establishment way ahead of the needs of the patient, of mistreating the symptoms, ignoring the body's messages—and making money while doing it.

Antibiotic side effects

Two of the most typical side effects of taking antibiotics are diarrhea and yeast infections, due to the suppression of our normal intestinal balance and the overgrowth of common yeast normally living in those intestines.

Taking antibiotics radically shifts the body's balance. Books such as *The Yeast Connection: A Medical Breakthrough* (William G. Cook,

Vintage Books, 1986) and *The Yeast Syndrome: How to Help Your Doctor Identify & Treat the Real Cause of Your Yeast-Related Illness* (Trowbridge and Walker, Bantam Publishing, 1986) describe the serious and growing problem of chronic mucocutaneous yeast infection, a debilitating and potentially fatal condition. One of the prime risk factors for chronic *candida* infection is repeated antibiotic use.

Our country's chronic cycle of antibiotic use, especially in this last generation, often begins in infancy, to treat ear infections or other common ailments that are usually accompanied by fever. Fever naturally occurs when our body is attacked by bacterial or viral infection; raising its temperature is our body's way of fighting off these infections. The important thing to understand here is that fevers happen for a reason and are NOT, as our society currently believes, inherently "bad."

In fact, fevers tell us exactly what is happening to our bodies when we most need to know. (Remember the temperature gauge in the car analogy?) Fevers are our body's signal that it's fighting off some kind of infection. In raising our body temperature, the fever is allowing our body to slow down the metabolic processes of the infectious organism, giving our immune system an advantage. It literally burns off the toxins, creates an unfavorable environment for bacterial and viral proliferation, and allows the body to cleanse itself.

However, when we take fever-reducing medication, we are undermining our body's inherent knowledge and ability to heal itself (what chiropractors call the body's "innate intelligence").

Innate intelligence is a way of respecting the body's natural processes. It says that when we get a cut, for example, our body knows just how to mend it and lay down new, healing tissue. When a bone breaks, our body inherently knows how to fuse it together and create new bone. We can use—and may require—stitches or a cast to make these injuries heal more quickly or to make the end result more attractive, but it is our innate intelligence that heals—and that wants to heal in the way it knows it should.

Yet another example of how our immune system's innate intelligence works is the cells in our body. Did you know that cancer cells constantly appear in our bodies? They appear on a regular basis, but our immune system immediately prevents them from growing or multiplying any further, ultimately killing them off. It is our immune system that has the ability to recognize abnormal cells through its innate intelligence.

With a fever, the body's innate intelligence knows exactly what it's doing when it raises our temperature to fight infection. Bringing the fever down prematurely by taking NSAIDS (anti-inflammatory agents) is like spreading apart a cut that has begun to heal and inviting a worse infection to take hold. We all know what happens if we do that: The cut will get inflamed, become infected and then, surely, you'll have no other option but to go on the antibiotics you wouldn't have needed in the first place if you'd let the cut run its course and let the body do what it knows so well how to do.

As a parent, of course, it's very hard to see our children suffer with a fever. They're tired, they don't look like themselves, they ache, and they may be crying. We think we're helping our child when our first line of defense is aspirin or baby Tylenol. But bringing a fever down automatically does not help our children; we're simply putting a band-aid on the symptoms to alleviate our natural concerns for their well-being.

In reality, bringing a fever down with drugs only makes things worse.

Letting your child's fever run its course will initially cause things to appear that they might be getting worse—but the achy feelings that often accompany a fever will not worsen the condition and often bring about the anticipated healing. On his Website, www.drlwilson.com, Lawrence Wilson, MD, notes that fever helps the body "burn up" toxins. As long as the infection process is controlled, it can actually be very useful, and using antibiotics to stop it prematurely can impair recovery in the long run.

Treating just the *fever* is the same kind of mistake as addressing only the end-stage result of a weakened body chemistry (bacterial invasion), when the body is too weak to eliminate the poisons that exist, or pulling out the tonsils to stop sore throats. These scenarios speak to the chiropractic philosophy of not treating a *symptom* that has manifested, but rather treating the *cause* of that symptom.

The bottom line here is that healthy people do not get as many infections, and infections do not strike randomly. Infections have a logic all their own, based on underlying causes that need to be addressed *before* they reach a more critical stage.

When is fever a good thing?

My area in South Florida was just recently hit by a nasty virus that caused fevers and, in some cases, vomiting and diarrhea. Every child in the area got it. All of my wife's friends were calling to tell her that their children were sick with fevers and, for the most part, these fevers had "turned into strep," ultimately requiring antibiotics.

Each child had one thing in common: their parent(s) tried to bring the fever down with NSAIDS. Their sickness ended up lasting six to eight days and all of them "required" antibiotics. In our family, the virus was handled differently.

My wife brought my oldest, Tyler, who already had a fever, into my office for an adjustment. Afterwards, I told my wife to give him plenty of water when they got home. That night his fever spiked and got as high as 104.2 degrees. But I was sure of the same thing I'm telling you here: that his innate intelligence knew what it was doing and I trusted in that. Ultimately his illness lasted all of fifteen hours and he was as good as new, without antibiotics and without a lengthy illness.

Thank goodness for fevers

In another case in which profits have come before true health care, the makers of NSAIDs (Advil, Tylenol, Naproxen, Motrin, etc.) claimed with consummate assurance that fevers are detrimental to our health to the degree that we need drugs to offset their effects.

In actuality, we know that fevers are a completely normal line of defense that the body draws upon when fighting some sort of sickness. I recently watched a show on the National Geographic channel on bees and hornets in Japan, and was struck by the parallel that could be made to our own systems when they are "under attack."

When under attack by a hornet, the bees have been found to surround the hornet in a "dense ball," according to the National Geographic Website (www.news.nationalgeographic.com/news/2007). The vibration of their bodies raises the hornet's temperature and forces it into heat stroke. Scientists studied how, when Cyprian bees were invaded by hornets, they clustered around the hornets in order to raise the temperature inside the clump to 111 degrees Fahrenheit. The bees as a group heat themselves to a precise temperature, somehow knowing that the hornets will die at a high temperature only 2 degrees lower than the honeybees themselves.

If we apply this strategy (i.e., the bee's ability to raise its temperature to save its own life) to our own body's system, we can see how useful fevers can be to ward off "invading" illness or infection—and to raise it safely in nine times out of ten.

What happens when we get a fever?

Let's talk about the actual mechanics of what has to happen in order for our body to increase its own temperature. Keep in mind that the body is so gifted at maintaining its core temperature that it regulates that temperature, keeping it constant to a mere tenth of one degree.

With that said, if it's generally agreed that a temperature of 98.6 is "normal" for most people, how do we maintain that core body temperature on a regular basis—regardless of the temperature outside our bodies?

On hot days, our bodies react by perspiring. Sweating is the body's way to moisturize the skin and cool down. On cold days, we shiver. Shivering is an activity akin to exercise—we are "working" our bodies in order to keep them warm. (This action is quite similar to what the honeybees do to generate enough heat to kill invading hornets.)

In an extreme condition such as being in excessive heat for a long period of time without enough water, our protective mechanism ultimately cannot produce the sweat we need. When it shuts down, we run the risk of suffering from dehydration and heat stroke. Normally, however, we have the ability to stay hydrated and rest, and our body automatically knows to regulate itself. We don't consciously have to tell it, "It's hot today. My body temperature is rising. Start sweating!" It inherently knows what to do to cool itself off.

The problem is that when our body temperature goes high enough, we interpret that not only as a sign of sickness, but as part of the sickness itself. In fact, medical manufacturers have tricked us into believing that the fever *is* the cause or is the actual illness itself, and that when we bring down the fever, we are no longer sick. So, by bringing a fever down artificially with NSAIDs, we're blocking our own body's pathway toward killing off the bacteria or virus—often causing a secondary bacterial infection in the lungs and ears.

Just two nights ago my four-year-old son had a fever of 101. He had a productive cough (coughing is the body's way of removing foreign material or mucus from the lungs and upper airway passages or of reacting to an irritated airway, and a productive cough produces phlegm or mucus in order to achieve this goal). We did the standard adjustment, rinsed his nasal passages with saline, and monitored his situation. I checked his temperature every half hour and, since it was stable at about 101, went to bed.

The next morning, my son woke up with a temperature of 98.5 and no cough or runny nose whatsoever. I know from my own experience and that of others that if we had brought down his fever artificially with NSAIDs, his condition would have worsened by morning. If that happened, he would have ended up at the doctor's with a prescription for antibiotics.

It's true that our kids have had fevers spiking as high as 104 on a number of occasions, which is relatively common with younger children. It is pretty easy, however, to offset rising temperatures with cool washcloths to the forehead and tepid baths, and to prevent dehydration by adding many extra fluids. Besides giving our kids an adjustment, we are diligent about making sure they drink as much water as they can. This brings the fever down much faster.

Of course, there are times when NSAIDs are important helpers, such as when the child is intolerably miserable from bodily aches and pains that occasionally accompany fevers. In that case, we avoid giving our children medication until the evening (on very rare occasions) to help them sleep. However, these occasions are rare because we know that such medication will cause their illness to last considerably longer than it has to.

To the body, a fever is a normal response when invaded by a virus or bacterial infection—it is an act as natural as breathing.

Giving a child NSAIDs to artificially bring the fever down is like holding him underwater, not allowing him to breathe—in other words, not allowing his body to do what it is naturally meant to do.

What about spinal meningitis?

One of the questions I hear a lot is, "What if my child's fever means something dangerous, like spinal meningitis?"

"Meningitis" is a term used to describe an inflammation of the membranes that surround the brain or spinal cord. This inflammation is normally a result of either a bacterial or viral infection (although other very rare causes are possible). It can also be caused by the direct spread of a nearby severe infection, such as an ear infection or a nasal sinus infection, and it often results in fever, lethargy, and a decreased mental status (obviously difficult to ascertain in a young child).

Meningitis occurs most often between the time of birth and two years of age, with the greatest risk immediately following birth and at three to eight months. Encephalitis, or inflammation of the brain, occurs if the infection or resulting inflammation progresses past the membranes of the spine or spinal cord.

If a parent is concerned that meningitis is a possibility, then it is conceivable that bringing the fever down artificially with NSAIDs could mask the very symptoms we would need to see in order to know there is a problem! The false sense of security we experience when our child's fever goes down might be the very thing that leads us to make the wrong decisions about his health.

On the other hand, there are certain symptoms that tip us off to severe illness—other than a relentless fever: (1) The child stops eating and/or drinking in the extreme; (2) The child has a stiff neck and is in pain; (3) The child is vomiting; and (4) The child's eyes hurt when looking at bright lights. Though rare, if any of these symptoms do present themselves, do not hesitate to bring your child to a physician or hospital emergency room.

How to help your sick child

There are ways to actually *help* the immune system in its function to fight illness:

- Always consider having your child adjusted immediately. This can alleviate many symptoms of illness, as well as correcting the cause of the symptoms.
- Use a saline lavage in nasal passages and aspirate out with a bulb syringe. Saline lavages slow down post-nasal drip, allowing the cough to go away usually in about a day. Additionally, saline soothes the irritated sinuses and creates an unfavorable environment for bacterial growth.

SALINE LAVAGE:

Have your healthcare professional demonstrate how to perform this on your child if you've never done it before. For children, use 2 tablespoons of salt per 1 gallon of distilled water. Inject ½ ml. in one nostril and ½ ml. in the other nostril. If mucus is brought out with the syringe, repeat the process.

In 90% of croupy, gurgly coughs, if you hear mucus coming up, it's probably just post-nasal drip. Inflamed tissues in the throat/pharynx make the trachea smaller in diameter. With added mucus, that area is condensed even more. Coughing forces a lot of air through a decreased hole and that's what produces the sounds. (If the cough goes into the child's lungs, there may be cause for concern, so always have a healthcare professional listen to breathing to ascertain if there is a secondary infection in the lungs.)

For adults, use 1/8 tsp. salt in 7 oz. of water. Cup the water in the palm of your hand and put your hand to your nose. Tilt your head back and allow the water to enter the nostril. You should be able to cough up the water that went into your nose and spit it out of your mouth, along with a lot of mucus.

Let's talk colds

In fact, let's talk colds, sinuses, and stuffy noses. And let's talk about what's real and what's not.

We've all heard, "Don't go outside without your hat because you'll catch your death of cold." Have you ever wondered if this was true, as you were stuffing your hat into your pocket as soon as you rounded the corner out of your mother's line of vision?

Though this particular myth has been debunked time and again, and holds no truth whatsoever, it still passes down from generation to generation. No one can deny that you'll be warmer with a hat and jacket, but it's certain that you won't "catch a cold" without them either.

A cold is actually a direct result of a viral infection, most commonly the rhinovirus. How are viral infections passed from person to person? Often by breathing in invisible droplets launched into the air by the sneezes of a person standing nearby. But extensive research has shown that these airborne droplets are not the only way the common cold is spread.

A significant source for transmitting colds is human contact. Cold viruses can survive up to three hours on a person's skin or on objects we touch, such as a book or faucet. We can transfer our cold germs—or get the germs of others—by shaking hands or turning on the faucet then using our hands to rub our eyes or bite our nails or wipe our mouth. The key here is washing our hands, of course. The more regularly you wash your hands after contact, the better off you are.

Here in Florida, people are always surprised when they get a cold because it's not cold outside. But the truth is that, although they actually do get "sick," it's not because they caught a viral infection at all. I have found that one reason people are more susceptible to certain "cold-like" symptoms is because they're constantly going from an outside temperature of above 90 degrees to an indoor temperature of 70 degrees set by air conditioners.

What are really causing these symptoms are their sinuses, which are extremely sensitive to drastic temperature changes. The sinuses are very thin membranes that react to temperature changes by secreting mucus as a defense. That's why symptoms such as a runny or stuffed-up nose appear. What these people are really experiencing is merely an excess of mucus as a direct result of their sinuses doing what they're supposed to do—protect themselves.

But therein lies the problem. In giving our sinuses a green light to protect themselves the only way they know how, we also create a perfect environment for bacteria and viruses to flourish. For all intents and purposes, our noses turn into petri dishes.

In a laboratory setting, if we wish to grow bacteria or viruses, we use a dish that contains an agar—a nutrient-rich, friendly environment in which organisms grow big and strong. Then the dish is placed in a nice, warm 98-degree oven to encourage growth. Sound familiar? Mucus is like fly paper to unwanted organisms floating around in the air. Normally, when we breathe these organisms in, our immune systems quickly extinguish them. But when there is excess mucus around, these organisms get trapped and that mucus becomes a breeding ground for viruses and bacteria.

Kids, antibiotics and the environment

Kids are growing up fast these days. Girls, in particular. In fact, girls are developing and menstruating earlier and earlier and in higher numbers, sometimes as soon as elementary school.

Not only that, it seems our kids, in general, are sicker than ever before. How is this possible, with all medical advancements we have made? Well, one of the most deleterious culprits is the food we ingest, which is full of steroids, antibiotics and vaccines. They get there through the same steroids, antibiotics and vaccines that are injected into our animals to make them grow more quickly and produce more. It's no coincidence: animals are growing faster and so are our children!

I consider this a literal epidemic, one that contributes not only to unprecedented growth and rushed development of our children, but to ever-climbing levels of illness in our population at large.

The process is a relatively uncomplicated one, though powerful in its effect. Meat companies are committed to the highest, fastest possible profits, and that means turning little calves and baby chicks into gigantic specimens as quickly as they possibly can. When that animal is slaughtered or that dairy cow has been milked, and the meat or milk arrives in our home, we simply end up consuming the same steroids, antibiotics, and vaccines the cow or the chicken or the pig had ingested.

Unfortunately, this scenario makes all too much sense in terms of the bottom line. If a farmer can spend a small amount of money on hormones and antibiotics and have a full-grown cow in half the time it would otherwise take, he's going to turn a profit much faster. Faster to grow, faster to the slaughterhouse, and faster to market.

The downside is that the consumer pays. And we pay with what we can least afford: our health.

How to reduce our need for antibiotics

There are two aspects to reducing antibiotic intake. The first is preventing infection by staying healthy, using proper hygiene to ensure cleanliness, exercising and getting the proper sleep, etc. The second is treating infections, when they do occasionally arise, with alternative methods.

Preventing infection requires a change in how we regard our environment. Drinking pure water and breathing clean air are just two of the ways to help our bodies stay strong. There are also many "green" products on the market now so that we can effectively throw away our toxic household cleaning agents while still keeping our surroundings clean.

We've already talked about a healthy diet to some extent, but certain nutrients (including vitamins A, C, E, selenium, and zinc) are powerful helpers for our immune systems. Fresh, organic, foods naturally contain much higher concentrations of nutrients than do the processed foods that comprise such large portions of our diets today. Again, hormone-free and antibiotic-free meats are also a critical part of a healthy diet.

Stress affects our bodies—negative thoughts and attitudes, fears, worries all tend to weaken our immune system, while positive thoughts can have amazingly beneficial effects. That's why meditation or deep breathing, which helps oxygenate the blood, can keep our immune system healthy, especially in times when stress becomes a factor.

In my practice, I often see patients arrive to my office in pain after having ignored symptoms that have been continuing for a significant length of time. Affecting a cure means approaching the real cause of the problem, and approaching it as early as possible. Many patients don't realize that their arthritic conditions are actually symptoms of an imbalance in the spine—and that imbalance is what needs to be addressed. In the case of infection, the same advice applies: Don't ignore the cause! If you do, even a simple cold, earache or cut can turn into a serious problem. Applying natural methods is the best way to ensure that that won't happen.

NSAIDs

Anti-inflammatories

One of the most prescribed treatments in our country is NSAIDs, or non-steroidal anti-inflammatory drugs. A common form is ibuprofen, and common brands include Advil and Motrin. Other forms of NSAIDS are aspirin, Nuprin, and Naproxin.

These drugs treat the symptom of inflammation, which is recognized as a type of nonspecific immune response. Inflammation is one of the ways in which the body reacts to infection, irritation, or other injury; its key features are redness, warmth, swelling, and pain.

There are so many signs of "inflammation" for which we now turn to NSAIDs—anything from headaches and backaches to cold symptoms. Curious about the seemingly all-encompassing attributes of these drugs, I asked my own friends and patients what they think happens when they take an Advil or Motrin for their pain. Their responses were similar: "It targets the pain. It goes right to it and deadens the irritated nerve." I have to admit to being surprised at these answers, although they did resemble the drug descriptions in the ads that we all hear: This product "goes right to the spot of your pain" and takes it away.

Sound familiar?

But reality is altogether different. I'm going to describe as simply as possible what really happens when we take one of these anti-inflammatories for pain.

Let's start with the pain itself. Where does it come from?

Pain is the body's signal that something isn't right, something "hurts." It sends this message via different internal pathways—what we can call "signaling paths." The path in particular that we're talking about here is the arachidonic acid cascade, which actually consists of more than twenty different signaling paths that control a wide array of bodily functions, but especially those functions involving inflammation and the central nervous system.

The role of the arachidonic acid cascade

The arachidonic acid cascade is one of the primary ways our body recognizes that inflammation—or pain—is present.

Most arachidonic acid in the human body is derived from dietary "essential fatty acids"—acids our body cannot produce on its own, but rather must come from dietary sources that contain fats (such as steak, eggs, and many cooking oils). We need arachidonic acids to perform their functions but, just like other bodily systems, we need them to be present in a balanced way.

When we experience an inflammatory response, two other groups of dietary essential fatty acids (for example, those ingested from oily fish or derived from flax oil) serve to offset or soften the inflammatory effects caused by too much of the first type, the arachidonic acid. To put it another way, when we take in too little of these other types of essential fatty acids, we leave ourselves open for heightened inflammatory responses from too much arachidonic acid—which means too much pain.

Let's look at these fatty acids, which you may have been hearing about on television or from your health practitioner, in a little more detail. Has a friend recently told you he's taking omega-3s? Have you heard about the diet that emphasizes eating flax seed oil or salmon—a fish very high in natural omega-3 oil?

If you have, it's because these are the fatty acids our body usually needs more of—the ones which counteract high concentrations of arachidonic acid that cause inflammation. The difference is that arachidonic acid is derived from an omega-6, not an omega-3, fatty acid. Although we also need omega-6 fatty acids for many important, everyday biological pathways to function, excessive amounts upset the balance.

The majority of sources suggest that 1:3 is an optimal ratio for omega-3 to omega-6 fatty acids, and that the current typical American diet *has a ratio of around 1:16*. Is it any wonder that so many of us are experiencing imbalances in our pathways, including inflammation in many areas of our bodies?

In support of this theory is an article by A.P. Simopoulos, "The importance of the ratio of omega-6/omega-3 essential fatty acids" (*Biomedicine and Pharmacotherapy*, 2002 Oct; 56(8):365-79). In the article, Simopoulos asserts that Western diets are too low in omega-3 fatty acids and too high in omega-6 fatty acids. This combination has been known to lead to diseases such as cardiovascular disease, cancer, inflammatory and autoimmune diseases. It has also been shown that a low ratio can help to suppress illness.

Interestingly, the study also reports that a somewhat higher ratio of omega-3 to omega-6 can actually suppress inflammation in patients with rheumatoid arthritis or asthma, but a much higher ratio of 1:10 had adverse consequences. So, we can say that although excessive amounts of omega-6 fatty acids may have negative consequences, they do maintain many crucial biological pathways that sustain our lives, including maintaining our stomach and intestinal linings.

If high amounts of arachidonic acid, a precursor to omega-6 fatty acids, increase the likelihood of both inflammatory and autoimmune conditions, how does this acid also maintain the lining of our stomachs? What happens is this: arachidonic acid enters the arachidonic acid "cascade," where it is transformed into chemicals called prostaglandins through the use of the enzyme cyclooxygenase, or COX. In other words, the COX enzyme converts arachidonic acid into prostaglandin—and when this COX enzyme is inhibited by drugs, we can experience relief from symptoms of inflammation and pain.

Of the two types of COX—COX-1 and COX-2—the first is crucial for maintaining the mucosal lining of our "gut" and regulating body homeostasis (balance). When we use a synthetic drug such as an NSAID to "turn off" that enzyme's reaction, we are also turning off the enzyme's ability to regulate our body's balance, particularly relative to our stomach and intestinal lining. When COX-1 is shut down, the mucosal lining disappears, leading to increased stomach acid, which results in bleeding ulcers. That's why so many people who stay on long courses of NSAIDs ultimately have ulcers; over time, the NSAIDs shut down the ability of arachidonic acid to transform appropriately and support our stomach's lining.

When COX-2 drugs such as Celebrex and Vioxx entered the market, they were welcomed with open arms by medical professionals and consumers alike. In targeting (shutting down) only the COX-2 sites, the stomach's integrity and the intestinal lining would be left uncompromised. But a problem occurred. The COX-2 targeted drugs were found to change the formation of prostaglandin—hence causing an increased risk for stroke and heart disease.

So the upshot on NSAIDs to treat inflammation is that side effects do occur, and some of them can be drastic.

That's why the real answer lies in maintaining a balanced ratio of omega-3 (the "good" fatty acids) to omega-6 (the "bad in excessive amounts" fatty acids), in order to avoid symptoms of aches, pains, inflammation and autoimmune conditions. When the ratio stays in check, everything works as planned.

To stay balanced naturally, we need to watch our intake of omega-6 fatty acids, which come in the form of animal fats, fried food, etc. Eating too many can easily increase our ratio to 1:15, with obvious negative results. In response, our body will attempt, as it always does, to self-balance, aiming for a ratio of 1:3. It does this by attempting to use up the store of omega-6 fatty acids by driving the arachidonic acid cascade forward once again. That is why limiting our intake of certain fats while increasing our intake of other healthy fats (from fish, flax, etc.) can help us alleviate many significant health issues, oftentimes altogether.

There are also alternative therapies to treat symptoms of inflammation. One is bromelain, an enzyme present in all parts of the pineapple plant and first introduced as a therapeutic supplement in 1957. According to *Medicine Plus* (www.nlm.nih.gov/medlineplus), it is classified as an herb and is said to help digest proteins when taken with meals. On an empty stomach, it is believed to work as an anti-inflammatory agent. In 1993, a panel approved bromelain to treat swelling of the nose and sinuses due to injury or medical procedure.

Bromelain has been used to treat a number of medical conditions, and is said to work by blocking some inflammatory metabolites that accelerate and worsen the inflammatory process. As an anti-inflammatory agent, it has been used for sports injury, trauma, arthritis, and other kinds of swelling, as well as for digestive problems, phlebitis, sinusitis, and healing after surgery. Bromelain is not only very easy to purchase, but easy to put through a juicer and drink. Nutri-West also produces a bromelain product, which I personally take.

To keep your intake of "good" essential fatty acids stable, I also recommend that both adults and children take fish oil capsules (DHA/EPA) daily for all kinds of symptoms, such as growing pains, muscle contusions, and bone injuries. If symptoms are not related to another kind of imbalance in the body that requires attention from an acupuncturist or chiropractor, they often respond well to the use of increased omega-3 fatty acids.

Antibiotics are not always the answer

Since natural remedies abound, it is generally a good idea to avoid antibiotics and NSAIDS—*and* their potentially dangerous side effects—whenever possible. If all it takes to cure your or your child's ills is a simple dietary change, isn't that the better way to go?

Many of my patients come to my office for an adjustment and, in the course of their appointment, tell me that their baby is on antibiotics for one reason or another. "My baby has strep throat again and had to go on amoxicillin" or "My baby has another ear infection and had to go on antibiotics again."

I cringe each time I hear these statements, knowing that some-times these tiny children are on constant courses of antibiotics. Can you imagine the possible effect on their immune systems' ability to fight off future bacteria? I also cringe because I know that 99% of the time antibiotics are not the appropriate treatment.

How do I know that? Because antibiotic treatment is seen as a way to achieve an immediate "fix" for something that probably needs a longer-term, natural response.

Many of us have experienced the situation when we start on an antibiotic and it seems to be helping, but then it stops doing its job and we need to start another course of a different kind. In this way, not only are we not giving our immune system the chance to work through whatever problem is occurring, we're also actually inhibiting it from doing its job over the long term, the same way NSAIDS inhibit our body's inherent ability to balance and self-regulate.

The more antibiotics and anti-inflammatory medications we take, the less able we are to be helped by them and the more apt we are to look to them to fix the ill health we have as a result of us weakening our immune systems.

When you automatically give your child antibiotics, you are not giving his or her immune system the chance to fight off whatever currently needs fighting off; you are also jeopardizing your child's health later in life. Immune systems need to be used in order for them to stay functional and healthy, or their ability to perform slows down over time.

Long-term antibiotic use (or short-term multiple use throughout a person's life) sufficiently weakens our immune system so that, when the time comes that we really need it to rally, it's no longer capable. That's one reason many people who enter the hospital for treatment of a particular illness have little resistance to the other bacteria present there. Elderly people or others with chronic diseases become targets for infections, such as pneumonia, because their immune systems are already in significantly weakened states after years of taking antibiotics and/or other medications.

Most people in the medical profession just prescribe "simple" antibiotics or NSAIDS and don't speak about the immune system this way. But I am a fervent believer that just as the heart must have nutrition and exercise, so must our immune systems. Give it a workout by letting it take care of lesser aches and pains and non-life-threatening illnesses, and help it out by eating healthily and balancing your body's intake.

Doctors prescribe endless courses of antibiotics for us and for our children. In this case, we shouldn't simply stay the course! When we use vaccines, NSAIDS, and antibiotics, we are virtually abusing our immune systems, the very system we need to stay intact. What happens to a heart that doesn't get exercise? It's not a healthy heart. If we let antibiotics fight all the battles of the immune system and suppress fevers when the body is performing a necessary function, the result is a sick immune system that turns into a *dysfunctional* immune system—one that causes sickness and cancer cell rates to elevate.

In the end, that dysfunctional immune system is what keeps the current, symptom based medical establishment flourishing. Remember, with our current medical system, in order for medical doctors to stay busy, we must stay sick.

CHAPTER SIX

HOPE

Genetics

In his book *The Biology of Belief: Unleashing The Power Of Consciousness, Matter, And Miracle* (Mountain of Love/Elite Books, 2005), former medical school professor and research scientist Dr. Bruce Lipton cites a study performed by Duke University that claimed healthy living can override genetic mutations in mice.

It seems that the pregnant mice in the study had an abnormal gene that caused severe obesity, and hence predisposed them to cardiovascular disease, diabetes, and cancer. These mice were given four supplements, which included vitamins B-9 and B-12, choline and betaine, all of which could easily be found at a health food store. Interestingly, the mothers that received the supplements gave birth to *standard, lean babies, even though their offspring had the same atypical gene.*

The mothers that did not receive supplements produced offspring that ate much more and weighed almost twice as much as the leaner ones. Furthermore, even though the offspring from both mothers were genetically the same, the heavier offspring (without natural supplements) were diabetic, while the lighter ones (with supplements) had no sign of diabetes.

This study makes it clear that genetic predisposition is only part of the puzzle when it comes to good health. Those of us who have diabetes that "runs in the family," or other medical or physical propensities, can take heart right now! This landmark study found that healthy living through supplementation actually overrode the mice's "genetic destiny."

I think about my patients who have children with asthma. They were told it was "in the child's genes"—that the natural inclination to have asthma could not be offset by anything besides asthma medication. What we need to realize is that respecting the five factors of health will give our bodies the best chance at true health, regardless of genetic predisposition. (In the case of children with asthma, I usually recommend that parents give them omega-3 fatty acid supplementations in addition to making sure they eat a healthy diet.)

Dr. Lipton further asserts in his book that "only 5% of cancer and cardiovascular patients can attribute their disease to heredity." That's an amazing statement, one with which I tend to agree. We are doing ourselves a disservice by spending so much time, energy and money studying genetics when we could be focusing on how to make the positive changes we need to make now.

Positive changes in our lifestyles and improving our environment at home and at work will help us find the positive mental attitudes we need to achieve optimal health. When talking about ways to stay healthy, we need to return to our discussion about what to avoid: drugs and their side effects. With their prevalence in the marketplace, on our shelves and in our lives, there is just no way to ignore the topic.

There is no drug available on the market without side effects—and the fact that most of the time we don't feel those side effects is a very frightening thought in itself. When we take a drug, it automatically has systemic effects; that is, it travels throughout our entire body. The drug targets a specific receptor but, as Dr Lipton stated, we have similar receptor sites throughout the body. When the drug interacts with the intended receptor site, we may see a decrease in our symptoms. However, similar receptor sites in other parts of the body, which have been functioning properly and should not be altered, are also targeted and are sure to be corrupted.

The side effects are so numerous from these drugs that if we were not specifically informed about the symptoms we may experience, we could go years with headaches, stomachaches or just general malaise without associating these conditions with the drug.

When I hear, "My doctor ran MRIs, CTs and everything is normal; now they have me on [whatever drug is being prescribed to offset the new symptoms]," I want to jump up and down in frustration. Patients tell me, "I have to get off these medications. I'm not myself; I feel like I have no emotion and I'm tranquilized all day." That's the drugs targeting things that shouldn't be messed with!

I have helped alleviate many patients of not only their primary symptoms (for which they were taking the original drug) but now their secondary symptoms, too. There are always patients who refuse to stop using alcohol or smoking, and even with regular adjustments, sometimes simply cannot seem to affect a truly changed, healthier, lifestyle. In those cases, we have to help as best we can by suggesting they consider the appropriate changes. The same thing now applies to those patients on a constant course of prescription drugs.

When drugs are the wrong thing to do

In the introduction to this book, I shared the email I sent to my friends and family about my son Nicholas' birth and subsequent hospitalization. You know that the nurses told us we would probably need to keep him on Prilosec "for at least six months" for his acid reflux.

Putting aside all the issues related to whether the diagnosis of acid reflux (inflammation/ulcers of the stomach and/or duodenum) was in fact a correct one, and also putting aside for the moment how a drug like this might affect him in the future, it's a real challenge for me to think that a newborn would require such a powerful drug as Prilosec in the first place.

I think back to how my wife and I stood there frightened, listening to the doctors and nurses telling us our newborn son would need to be on drugs for many months, and I know without a shadow of a doubt that had I not myself been aware of the dangers of drugs on the human body, had I not known of alternatives for alleviating potential conditions such as the one from which my son was suffering, had I had not known chiropractic…I would have done exactly what the medical staff suggested. Who knows what the consequences would have been?

But I did know. And the amazing reality is that after my son's adjustment, he did not need Prilosec—or any other drug. Not only would the Prilosec have merely covered up a symptom of something that required fixing, he could have been severely damaged by side effects from the drug.

Furthermore, the "diagnosis" was based on symptoms, not the actual cause of that symptom, which was a bone in the spine that had rotated out of its correct position. This rotated bone caused an imbalance that caused a dysfunction—misalignment—that then irritated the nerve. The effect of this misalignment meant a dysfunction of some kind was inevitable, whether the nerve ultimately led to the stomach or the lungs. Medication would have done nothing more than temporarily mask the actual root problem.

Prilosec is a strong drug that causes a decrease in the acidity of the stomach. That can lead to another, two-fold problem because we need our stomach acid to naturally break down what we eat, and decreasing acidity automatically throws the acid levels of the stomach off balance. A certain level of acidity must be maintained: A healthy stomach has an acidity level (pH) between 1 and 2, around one million times more acid than pure water. The digestive process takes place as food passes through the mouth, stomach, small intestine and large intestine. At the stomach, the gastric acid helps to break down proteins for further digestion at the small intestine.

Let's look at a good comparison. Have you ever heard the phrase, "An acid neutralizes a base"? Think of the typical swimming pool. To keep a pool clean, you occasionally have to add acid called muriatic acid, also known as hydrochloric acid. It's so strong that it would burn layers upon layers off your skin if you came in contact with it. The opposite of a strong acid is a strong base, which is very caustic as well (an example of one is a commercial drain cleaner). A strong base is usually sodium hydroxide, also known as lye or caustic soda.

If these two extremely strong compounds are added together in the correct amounts, they cancel each other out to form a solution that's as neutral and harmless as water. So why do I use the examples of a pool and a drain cleaner? Because when we eat, the contents in the stomach are very strongly acidic. On the other hand, the chemicals inside the small intestines are strongly basic. When the contents of the stomach empty into the small intestines, an acid meets a base and things neutralize so they can proceed through the rest of our digestive system the way nature intended.

When we alter the acidity, or pH, by using a drug like Prilosec (which lowers the amount of acid in the stomach), we are likely creating other potential problems that could create long-term consequences.

I'm going to continue on with Nicholas' story for the benefit of all new parents out there who may find themselves in such difficult and confusing circumstances.

At first we were sure that our baby just had too much milk and the result was an overfilled stomach that was causing him to vomit. That's what I suggested, many times over, when the nurses took our baby away from us and back to the nurses' station to be monitored. They assured me this wasn't the case, since they attempted to burp him (properly) with no luck and no relief.

At this point, our precious little two-day-old son was exposed to needle after needle, two stomach lavages (when a tube is inserted through the nose and into the stomach, pumping saline in and then aspirating it out), a lung x-ray to "rule out pneumonia," multiple x-rays while drinking barium out of a bottle, brain EEG studies, an echocardiogram on his heart, and more needles.

Nicholas' milk intake was monitored very closely and kept small, but his episodes of vomiting did not stop. The nurses even gave him rice mixed in with the milk, in an attempt to "weigh" the milk down in the stomach so it wouldn't come back up. Clever, but that didn't work either. Eventually the continuous vomiting resulted in a hypoxic condition (where the blood has inadequate amounts of oxygen), causing him to be given oxygen.

With the "too-much-milk" theory ruled out, the hospital staff struggled to find an answer. When every test came back negative and no one could explain why our son was experiencing problems so severe, he was admitted to the ICU. He was subjected to even more tests, all of which were negative, but was still vomiting as well as suffering from hypoxia, which required supplemental oxygen. After around two days, he was put on antacids and proton pump inhibitors. "By default," they told us, "it must be acid reflux."

After several treatments of his acid reflux "cocktail," they said we would be able to take him home the next morning, but another episode of vomiting and loss of breath did not allow for that. We were then told he would need to stay in the ICU for a minimum of forty-eight more hours—or until they figured out the cause of his symptoms. The doctor wanted to change the "cocktail."

We were desperate. We agreed.

Doing what you feel is right
During his few first days of life, before ever being admitted to the ICU, Nicholas was examined by a pediatric cardiologist, a pediatric neurologist, a pediatric respiratory specialist, and a pediatric gastrointestinal physician.

These specialists were extremely bright, caring, and kind, and if my son had a legitimate medical need for one of them, I wouldn't think twice about utilizing their services. We felt comfortable with them and their competence; we just couldn't reconcile the fact that every one of them was telling us that although each part of our baby's body was functioning normally, he was still having such major health issues.

When we were told that the lung x-ray was to rule out pneumonia, our question was: How can a two-day-old infant have pneumonia? What does that possibility say about the hospital environment? Then, when we were told his blood test showed "banding," or possible infection, we wondered how that would even be conceivable in a "good" hospital with a safe, sterile environment.

Then I remembered… Just after Nick was born, we were sitting in our room waiting to hold him. I went to wash my hands in the adjoining bathroom and couldn't believe my eyes when I saw raw sewage coming up through the drain in our sink! Mortified, my wife and I filed a complaint with the hospital but it took three separate filings to get the problem fixed. The maintenance man told us that someone else's toilet had backed up, causing similar backups in other people's rooms that were connected to the same line—including ours.

Needless to say, I had expected a better plumbing system in what we had felt was a reputable hospital, and we felt sick about the possibility that our son had become the victim of such potentially dangerous circumstances. I told the nurse that we had reported the problem three times and it still had not been repaired and asked how it was possible that a hospital caring for a newborn could allow such a thing to happen.

That's when things really went south.

There was no change in his status at this point, so Nick was taken to the nursery to monitor him more closely.

There, we asked a lot of questions of the nursing staff but were met with abrupt answers. Something was wrong with our child, and we just wanted to know that we were in a friendly, caring place. I felt helpless.

I would walk over to the nursery and wait patiently until a nurse was available to ask how my son was doing. It seemed like a simple question, but I had to fight to maintain my composure and not break down completely right there in the hospital hallway each time I asked it. The answers I received were short: "Your son's not doing well. We had to give him oxygen because his blood oxygen levels dropped. We need time to figure things out. We'll come get you when we know more…" They said this with so little compassion, and sighed as if we were bothering them.

In desperation, we called our own pediatrician to try to better understand what was happening. We had chosen this particular hospital because it was closer to our home than the one where our pediatrician had staff privileges, not realizing how much of a difference that would make. Although she was technically the baby's physician, she wasn't able to come and offer her expertise. The best she could do was ask us to find out from the nursing staff certain test results so that she could interpret them and, hopefully, put our minds at ease.

I wrote down everything she wanted to know then Janice and I walked to the nursing station. When I asked one of the nurses if I could get the information our pediatrician needed, she responded with, "What??" and a sigh. Then she told us to "hold on" while she went to get another nurse. The new nurse walked out…and I'll never, ever forget what happened next.

I remember how this woman looked, her build, her demeanor, everything. She glanced at us then said, her face stern and unemotional, "You both need to come with me. I need to speak to you and your wife in private."

I looked at Janice, she looked at me, and we both started to cry. We were certain she was going to tell us that our son had died. I felt that I was going to faint; my legs felt heavy, my heart felt like it was being crushed, I couldn't breathe. I kept saying to myself, "Stay strong, Scott, please stay strong for Janice…just hold it together for her." I fought against a complete breakdown with as much inner strength as I could muster.

We made it to the hospital room where the nurse told us to have a seat, pointing to the chairs. I could tell that Janice was about to pass out; she was as white as a sheet. I held her hand, waiting for the bad news. The nurse stood there, towering over us, and said, "You can't keep coming over and asking us these questions about your son. Your pediatrician has no staff privileges at this hospital, so we can't give any information out."

Janice and I were confused but silent. Unbelievable as it was, we were being denied the information we requested—about our son!!

Then the nurse said, "Have you ever heard of HIPAA? Sharing that information would violate HIPAA laws." HIPAA is the Health Insurance Portability & Accountability Act put in place in 1996, which deals with privacy regulations. "The information you're asking about is private and is not intended for any third parties, so you need to let us do our job."

The one thing I knew right then was that this was no time for a discussion about insurance! I went from nearly fainting to fuming. I jumped up out of my chair and yelled, "HIPAA?! My son is sick and you brought us here to talk about that? I thought you were going to tell us that he died!!"

Up until that point, through extreme self-control, I had been quiet, polite, and composed through the whole experience. I said, "Are you sure you want to go down that HIPAA road with me!? You'd be making a huge mistake. I've already noticed at least five violations on this floor." And I really had.

I focused on her eyes and glared at her directly, never losing contact. Then I said it again: "Are you sure you want to take that road, because I will file complaints right now!"

By this time, the nurse was shaking. I looked down at her hands and they were visibly shaking. She said slowly, "Are you a doctor?"

I said, "Yes, but that doesn't matter here. I want to know what's wrong with my son."

She just about crumbled and immediately apologized for her actions. Still, we didn't know what to do. Our son was very sick, and we had no answers.

A few hours after Janice calmed down, I took a ride back to our house, where I proceeded to contact my mother's best friend, the chief administrative officer of a well-respected hospital. She told me what I had already suspected—that it was our right to access any information we wanted regarding our child. Furthermore, it was my right to pass that information on to my pediatrician.

As soon as I put down the phone with my mother's friend, I picked it up again to call the administrator of the hospital where my son was, and was put in contact with the nursing administrator. I let her know what had transpired with the nursing staff, how they had refused to provide information about my son's condition, and I also told her about the sewage problem I had reported three times. As I talked, I started to cry, overwhelmed by the situation.

The nursing administrator assured me that it was our right to have the information we wanted and that, although our pediatrician wasn't treating our child in the hospital, she had the right to decipher test results. Then she indicated her dismay that Janice hadn't been moved from that room with the sewage problem, apologized, and said she'd do her best to make sure the rest of our experience was "pleasant."

She personally went to Janice's room, had the nursing staff move her immediately into one without faulty plumbing, brought several gift certificates, and stayed to talk to Janice to make sure she was all right. She replaced our nursing staff and I never saw those same nurses again during our entire stay. Our new nurses were very kind and we felt the administrator was caring and sincere.

Unfortunately, though, Nick had reached the point where he had to be put into neonatal intensive care because his symptoms weren't diminishing.

The next day at the ICU, he was no better. He had an episode and had to be given more oxygen. We were so frustrated. I turned to Janice and said, "We've given the hospital and the doctors every chance. As a chiropractor, I know every nerve that goes to every organ that does everything in the body. Something must have been impeding something right from the start, right from Nicholas' birth process. If you believe in what I do, you'll agree to my adjusting our son right now."

Exhausted from the birth and emotionally drained by Nicholas' condition, she agreed without hesitation.

I waited until the nurses weren't watching. Then I put Nicholas on my lap, on his stomach, and gently adjusted his back. I adjusted him at the T6-7 level, where the nerves connect to the stomach, and we heard tiny "pops" in the thoracics and then a "pop" again. Suddenly, the baby was quiet. All his symptoms stopped. He didn't vomit, started to eat and became, once again, the perfect newborn.

The problem was gone—hence, the subtitle of this book, "A chiropractic miracle."

Nicholas' medical team insisted he had improved due to his newest drug "cocktail" but we knew better. They recommended he stay on the drugs for a minimum of six months.

When we received the bills from the hospital for the five days, they were in excess of sixteen thousand dollars.

We went back to our own pediatrician's office a short time later and I told her about the adjustment I'd done on Nicholas. I was concerned she'd be skeptical or have a negative reaction, so I waited anxiously to hear her response. She was completely supportive! Not only did she believe that what I'd done helped Nicholas, she also informed me about many of the things the hospital staff had done incorrectly (such as feeding him rice milk).

We came to a crossroads. Janice and I said we felt strongly about taking our son off the drug cocktail and would be taking him off all medications, a mere two days after leaving the hospital. Curious, we asked our pediatrician for her opinion. She agreed, adding that we should keep the medicine around in case his symptoms came back.

But they never did.

We even had to have a large heart and breathing monitor delivered to our home, per the hospital's instructions, to hook Nick up to every night before bed to warn us of any breathing problems that might be related to the vomiting issues he suffered from in the hospital. For the four months that we had him hooked up to the machine, the alarm never sounded one time, even though he was never given one drug.

It's quite amazing that one gentle little spinal adjustment could be so powerful in helping such a tiny body achieve health.

In contrast...

When our third child, Hannah Rose, was born, the experience was so vastly different from the one with Nick that I think it's important to include it here.

I'm so happy to be able to say that the entire experience with the birth of Hannah Rose was absolutely perfect. We went to a hospital called Mease Countryside in Clearwater, Florida. It was a bit of a drive, but our trusted pediatrician was on staff there and if we had any issues or complications, I wanted her to be presiding over all decisions.

Before the birth, I thought I was doing a good job of hiding my fear, but my office staff, who know me well, could see I was stressed. I was afraid of a repeat performance even though we had done everything humanly possible to make sure that didn't happen. We decided to do things very differently this time; we even had a birth plan, specifically listing what we expected that would make this an enjoyable experience for us.

At the other hospital, when we made small requests or had certain expectations, we were met with rudeness and dirty looks— "it's-our-way-or-the-highway" kind of looks. We felt as if we had given up all of our rights and were imprisoned until the baby was ready to leave the hospital. Of course, a few of the nurses were really pleasant but the majority had a negative vibe about them.

Mease Countryside was quite the contrast. When we handed the birth plan to the nurse, I gritted my teeth and thought, "Well, here goes—let's see how she reacts." The nurse smiled, started reading the list and said out loud, "Okay, uh-huh, looks good, good." Then she looked up at us cheerfully and said, "This is perfect. We can accommodate you on everything!"

I took the deepest, relaxing, most cleansing breath that I had taken in a long time. I knew right then and there that this would be a great experience…and it was! The nurses were so caring and efficient. Do you know that warm, positive feeling you get when you're around someone who you know deep down is genuinely kind? Both Janice and I felt that with every staff member at the hospital: the obstetrician/gynecologist, the anesthesiologist, the OR staff, everyone.

The experience was amazing. All the way, even through the recovery, the nurses were there for Janice, for me and for our daughter, providing a feeling of comfort. It's the first hospital where I have actually enjoyed staying.

Janice had purchased a whole bag of body lotions prior to going into the hospital. Assuming the nurses were kind, she planned on giving each of them a bottle of scented lotion as a gift for taking good care of us. Needless to say, we ended up wanting very much to share the gifts with the nursing staff, who were touched and thankful that Janice went out of her way to show her appreciation to them.

Giving makes you feel good. Most Christians, meditation experts and philosophers will suggest that you give without the expectation of gaining anything in return. We have to admit that it was a little tough for us to assume we would have a wonderful experience when the last one had been so dismal, so we were a bit selfish in waiting to see how it turned out before deciding to give the gifts. But we are so glad we made the effort, and I highly recommend buying something for the entire nursing staff that takes care of you during a hospital stay.

However, please don't expect the nursing staff to wait on you hand and foot—you're not at a five-star hotel, after all. Their job is to keep Mom and baby stable, nothing more. You have every right to expect to be treated with care and respect, but they do not have any obligation to cater to the father or other family members, only the mother and baby. Knowing that, I must say another thank you to Mease Countryside for going above and beyond in making our experience so wonderful.

Not all "Western" physicians are created alike

As the chiropractic treatment on my newborn son shows, I am a big believer in using the right tool for the job. That's why I avail myself of Western medicine as well as many other types of therapies.

That said, I feel obligated to comment on those aspects of the medical profession that give rise to concerns about its power and misuse, as well as to share the positive experiences I've had with members of the traditional medical establishment.

By now, you know how incredible my pediatrician is. Dr. Danuta Jackson-Curtis is worth her weight in gold, as are many other M.D.s with whom I've had the pleasure to work (such as Dr. David Boaz, whose interview is included in this chapter). It's very important that I communicate this fact because I don't want to denigrate all of Western medicine in an attempt to promote alternative treatments such as chiropractic.

To underscore that point, if our pediatrician were one hundred percent certain that my son needed to be on a specific medication, I would not only consider it, I would probably agree to it because—and only because—I know she is a believer that the body has great power to heal itself and that she uses medication only as a last resort. I have a great admiration for that belief.

I knew about our pediatrician's beliefs through her care of our first child, Tyler, but was reminded again one day when my second son, Nicholas, was about five weeks old. Nick had a very crusty eye on one side. We assumed the tear duct was blocked because, even though we cleaned it, thick, mucus-y secretions would reappear within two hours in and around his eye.

We went to the pediatrician's office and Dr. Jackson-Curtis took a look at it. I said unhappily, "We need to go to an ENT (Ear, Nose, and Throat physician) to have the tear duct unblocked, don't we?" She responded, "Absolutely not! That's a last resort." What she said next surprised me even more.

Her instructions were that, three to five times a day, we should use a dropper to put two or three drops of my wife's breast milk in Nick's eye, then massage the area bordering the lower eyelid on the side closest to the nose. She indicated that a mother's breast milk not only has natural lubricants in it, but it also has natural antibiotic characteristics. We did what she instructed and the crusty, caked-on discharge was completely eliminated in about four days *and never returned.*

As I've said, that is the power of natural healing—and that is the hope that true healthcare professionals can give us.

An Interview with Dr. David Boaz

Dr. David Boaz is another such healthcare provider who inspires hope in his patients and colleagues.

Flying home from Atlanta, where my family and I had stayed with Dr. David Boaz and his family, I found myself thinking how forty or fifty years ago—maybe even as recently as ten years ago—you would never have seen a chiropractor and a medical doctor sitting down together over a beer and a cigar, just to talk about life and health.

I met David Boaz when he referred a patient to me for care; after I sent a follow-up letter to discuss the patient's progress, we hit it off. Since then we've cultivated a great relationship. He's the perfect example of the kind of medical doctor I want people to see, someone open-minded, who cares about *you* first.

Dr. Boaz is very open to the benefits of chiropractic care, and when it comes to prescriptions, he thinks long and hard about the patient before writing one. We'd been talking about Vioxx and how, even before it was pulled from the market, he'd only written one prescription for it because he thought it was overpriced and didn't work as well as people said it did. To me, he's a real hero in the profession.

If I personally had to see a medical doctor, I would want to go to someone like him because if he told me to take a medication, I would believe I legitimately needed it. I wouldn't feel that way with most medical doctors.

Here is our interview:

DR. PATON: *When you got out of medical school, what were your thoughts in terms of alternative treatments and providers?*

DB: Basically when you go through medical school they teach you to treat with medications in a certain way. When you go through your rounds in medical school they teach you to practice in the way they've always practiced. And a lot of doctors don't practice any alternative methods so you wouldn't know…

To be honest, I never paid much attention to chiropractic. I'd heard doctors who looked down on chiropractors and I never really thought after I graduated medical school that I would ever refer to a chiropractor. If there were something musculoskeletal going on with the patient, I would refer to a physical therapist, prescribe a muscle relaxant or anti-inflammatory, and follow up with the patient. I never considered using a chiropractor.

It wasn't really until I got out into private practice and had patients who actually saw chiropractors and who told me they had a lot of benefit that I started reconsidering. Patient after patient had pain, surgeries, medications, but they never really got relief until they were adjusted—and then they got a lot of relief.

It took a while for me to realize the truth about something I hadn't considered, and to really understand that you have to do what's right for the patient, that you can't just treat by what the books say. And over time I found that you can work with chiropractic or acupuncture and still use medication, physical therapy, and everything else in conjunction to get the overall benefit for the patient.

It's one of the those things where you study something or you see something and you assume that's the only way to approach it, but over time, as you practice, you find out there are many ways to approach a situation. Every person responds differently. One person may respond well to medication or exercise therapy whereas another person may not respond at all.

Lately the medical profession in general has come to support chiropractic, especially in family medicine. If you look at some of the journals, there are a lot of articles on lower back pain, musculoskeletal symptoms, which include chiropractic, and you find that there is more and more support as the years go on and more and more evidence that manipulation does help.

DR. PATON: *After what happened to my Nick when we adjusted him in the hospital as a newborn, I would love to see chiropractors functioning inside the hospital to help in those kinds of situations.*

Since then, I've heard from so many new parents who have experienced similar circumstances, and who have complied with medical recommendations (directives, really) to keep their infants on drugs for long periods of time. For those situations where the doctors say, "Everything looks fine, but by default we're going to try this or this or this," I think parents deserve to have another option.

DB: I think medical doctors should rotate through chiropractic and through acupuncture to at least experience those during medical school and residency. I also think that chiropractors should have the opportunity to rotate through a medical physician's office to see how things are treated in different way. Because if you're accustomed to thinking there's only one way to treat something, you are not open to all the options every doctor should know.

I think physicians should learn about Asian medicine and what it has to offer, because when a patient comes in for help, they want to know about anything they can do to correct or improve their condition or general state of health. Patients don't get the same education that the physician in medical school is going to get. So it's important that the physician has as many options as possible to communicate to the patient.

DR. PATON: *I often think about how people listen to their doctors—go to them for advice and listen to what they say. You have to hope that these doctors know what they're talking about.*

For example, you're in good shape, David. I've said in this book that I would never take medical advice of any kind from a doctor who can't take care of him- or herself. There are people I see at the state association meetings who obviously take poor care of themselves, and I wonder how patients feel about taking their opinions to heart. I think I'm going to ruffle a lot of feathers by saying that, but what's your opinion?

DB: I found myself in a similar situation for a while. I was busy and, well, I got to the point where I wasn't exercising much and was often recommending that patients exercise though I wasn't doing it myself.

Finally I figured out that I needed to start taking care of myself and several years ago started an exercise program, which I have continued. I found that when you start practicing what you preach, it changes your attitude. You have a lot more confidence in recommending something if you've experienced it yourself. Whether it's being on a medication, doing an exercise program or a diet program, you can convey to the patient a whole lot better what you've been through, and the patient is more likely to follow the regimen, or at least understand the regimen, and be more compliant if he knows that the person recommending it has been through a similar experience.

DR. PATON: *When I interviewed a fitness consultant for this book, I asked him a question and I'd like to get your opinion on the same question, too. I used the example of the patients who have a hard time holding their adjustments because they're overweight. Due to the excess weight there's too much stress placed on their spines, and they're sway-backed because they're always trying to offset the weight in the front. I try to tell them that, although I'm glad I help them feel better, adjusting can only be a temporary fix, and until they fix the real problem they won't hold the adjustments. So I encourage them to begin exercise programs—walking, jogging, whatever they can do.*

But in my experience, most of them give up almost before they've begun. I know how hard it is to keep going when you first start out— when I've let myself get out of shape it's always a struggle to get back into shape—but I didn't understand why if I could push through the stage of wanting to give up, these patients could not. They come up with every excuse in the book—and I have, too. No matter what I do, though, I can't motivate them to keep going.

So what makes some people ignore the voices that tell them to quit, and some people decide to keep going? The personal trainer's response was that there are any number of psychological issues that are contributing to the person's weight problem to begin with, and issues that contribute to their being able to take the weight off. They have to get to the root of the problem enough to get the person to the next level.

What's your thought about this? Why is it so easy to quit when I'm telling them that they're wasting their money by not taking my advice?

DB: A lot of people want that quick fix. In today's world, it's hard to make the point that you have to take the time to take care of yourself. There are so many other things going on—a lot of it is genetic, a lot of it is lifestyle…you can get hooked on a certain lifestyle. And to a lot of people, exercise is not enjoyable. I exercise myself and have to admit I don't enjoy going to the gym myself, but once I finish I feel good.

The dentist tries to tell people to brush their teeth everyday and most people do, but only because they've learned from childhood and that's what they've always done, and they know if they don't do it their teeth may fall out. But I don't think physicians have done as good a job conveying to people how and why to live a certain lifestyle. Sometimes people have too little time between working and everything else they need to do—and eating is enjoyable. Exercise is not always enjoyable, especially initiating it, and people don't have the time, or feel as if they don't have the time.

DR. PATON: *So you think it's more of a lifestyle issue?*

DB: Well, I think it's a big issue. Once someone is motivated to try a different kind of lifestyle, they become more aware of their health.

DR. PATON: *My only question, then, is what about the people who continue to say, "I just can't, my knees hurt, I've tried…"? They've made the time but they're still overweight and miserable. I'll send them to the orthopedist, who sees nothing wrong…how do you get through to those people with the excuses? They might make the time, but don't get any further than that. Could it be emotional?*

DB: Definitely. There are so many factors that go into a person's life. I've run into a lot of people and emotional issues are affecting the way they take care of themselves. A lot of stress makes a difference. A quick fix—alcohol, eating more, sleeping more—seems easier. They don't want to take the time to take care of themselves.

Drive-through fast food is tasty and quick and a pretty good deal and you feel like you're eating something that makes you full. If you eat something healthy and exercise, it takes a much bigger portion of time out of your life. They don't realize that, in the end, you've saved time (and possibly your life) by making an investment in yourself. In America, the attitude of "buy this, buy that" to try to satisfy yourself as much as possible with material things really doesn't end up satisfying you in the long run. But in the meantime, you get the quick fix, like a drug, and go on to the next thing.

DR. PATON: *So how would you approach the person who needs help but, for whatever reason, can't get going with exercise?*

DB: In my job as an educator, I specifically tell people that I'm going to give them advice, but what they do with it is up to them. I see from my experience that if you are overweight, if you don't take care of yourself, if you smoke, if you drink, chances are you're going to end up with heart disease, cancer, maybe other diseases at an early age.

At first it doesn't seem to hurt a lot of people to be over-weight—it's not painful, at least early on. By the time it becomes painful, they're stuck with the lifestyle that made them that way. By then people are reluctant to change their attitudes and part of my job is to encourage and explain the benefits of changing behaviors and attitudes.

I think it's human nature to live for the day, not really think about tomorrow. Look at all the people who are in debt, spending more than they earn, more than they have. It's true from a medical standpoint, too. People don't often look at the future, at their poten-tial, but only at what they have now and what they can do now and what is easiest for them.

DR. PATON: *I want to switch gears and ask a question for all the chiropractors who read this book. Can you give me an example of how medicine saved someone's life? I'd like to remind all of us—including chiropractors—to be as open-minded as we'd like medical doctors to be. Does anything come to mind?*

DB: I can think of a lot of cases.... Medicine has evolved over many centuries; we don't just prescribe medications, and we're not all slaves to the drug companies. The doctor's main interest is to heal the patient, to make the patient feel better. And a doctor is going to go out of business if he prescribes whatever the drug companies put out. If that's what happens, the patients won't go back to that doctor, either. They have to be able to trust the doctor.

I remember once a patient came in and I was listening to her lungs. She was a heavy smoker, about a pack a day, a young person in her late 20s. You could hear wheezes and abnormal lung sounds. I remember telling her, "Your lungs sound horrible, like an old person's, and they're not living up to their full function."

We see a lot of smokers who say they're going to quit, but they don't quit; they come back smoking just as much. But this patient came back a few months later and said she remembered my talking about how bad her lungs sounded. She told me, "I thought about it and I quit smoking." She said there was something I said that got her to quit.

Looking back, that's one of the most rewarding things in medicine, beyond any finances or other rewards, when you can look back and say that there was something you did or said, however simple, that helped a patient make a change in their life that potentially allows them to live longer and healthier and have a more rewarding life. That's worth more than anything.

DR. PATON: *Have you ever found any type of cancer in a patient?*

DB: I have, several times. The patient might come in with a mild symptom—a small abdominal pain, for example—and we may do a CT scan and find a tumor. Often, once the tumor is removed and the patient has the cancer treated, he starts to look at his life with a totally different perspective. They begin to question why they got the cancer, maybe because they smoked or hadn't taken care of themselves, and sometimes they change their lives for the rest of their lives.

DR. PATON: *This relates precisely to the "five factors of health" as I lay them out in the book—as a lifestyle to stay healthy. A person's chances of staying healthy are much greater when they follow the five factors—enough exercise, enough sleep, a positive mental attitude, good nutrition, and ongoing chiropractic care. But because there are always environmental risks, either personal ones such as smoking, or external ones such as contaminated water or air pollutants, medical treatment provides the treatment and care people often need once symptoms have created certain conditions.*

That's why chiropractors also have to be open-minded and send their patients to good medical doctors when the situation arises. Chiropractors don't routinely look at the lungs or listen to the heart, for example. Both physicians and chiropractors need to work in partnership to provide the best service possible for their patients.

Unfortunately, I have to add also that sometimes we chiropractors send patients for tests or consultations to medical doctors who demean our profession to the patient. This is something we can only hope will improve over time. And, luckily, there are many doctors, like you, who do not behave in that manner. I can only say that in meeting you, I got lucky, because now I have someone to whom I can refer my patients when they need traditional medical attention.

DB: I don't believe there is any place in any type of medical practice for ego. There is a big difference between confidence and ego. It's good to have a doctor who's comfortable and confident in what h/she does, but who also understands that the human body is a lot more complex than everything he or she has learned.

I see this every single day in practice, that there are things that you are just not going to know. And there are things that other doctors are not going to know. You have to be of the mentality that you are treating the patient and not treating your own ego. There's no place for that attitude. You need to leave your ego at the door and ask, "What is best for this person? How can I make this person's life more rewarding? How can I help this person's symptoms improve and prevent further problems down the road?"

DR. PATON: And that's one thing I hope this book will restore— or build: trust between medical doctors and chiropractors.

DB: *Yes, I hope not only that chiropractors will begin to trust that there are doctors out there who will work with them, but that the doctors will also start looking at all ways possible to treat the patient. You have to have the attitude that if one thing doesn't work, you'll make every effort possible to find something that does work for the patient.*

And patients have to make an effort, too, to take care of themselves and do the right things, to explore all the avenues to find what will work. Many of the changes that need to occur need to occur outside the practitioner's office, in the life of the patient.

The other side of the coin

Both chiropractors and chiropractic patients need to appreciate medicine as much as I'm asking medicine to appreciate chiropractic.

We are so blessed to live in the United States because of the medical technology we possess. I couldn't think of a better place to be than an American hospital if I had acute injuries, say from an auto accident. Like I've said throughout this book, medicine in the United States treats the symptom, rather than the body, regarding *chronic* conditions. On the other hand, in *acute* conditions that are life threatening, the symptom may be low blood pressure due to a severed artery. In this case, of course, you'd want to treat the symptom—if you're going to save the person's life.

Therefore, I'm certainly not opposed to using medicine in some cases, but it's usually the acute cases for which medicine is most valuable. Chronic cases such as IBS, headaches, etc. that require people to be on a long-term medication regimen is where the U.S. is doing things backwards.

If you are a chiropractor or chiropractic patient, please don't disparage medicine; try to recognize the positive side. I once heard a chiropractor telling others about how bad medicine is, when a few months prior his son was treated by an orthopedic surgeon for a broken arm. I thought he was a hypocrite.

I believe, as Dr. Boaz said, that the way we should start to make a change for the better is to have medical doctors do rotations in a chiropractic office, and also have chiropractors do rotations in a medical setting. If this were the case, there would be a mutual respect for each profession.

Personally, I try to maintain professional relationships with medical doctors, acupuncturists, and physical therapists. It's so nice to be able to confidently refer people when they need care beyond the scope of what I can do in a chiropractic setting.

I used to perform basic sports rehab in my office. As my practice got busier, I only had time to do chiropractic, so I started referring patients to a physical therapist down the street named Jill. Jill and her co-workers have done an excellent job on every patient that I've referred to them. We have lunch on occasion and it gives me a chance to explain chiropractic and them a chance to explain what they do regarding therapy.

In cases such as these, the patient always wins, because they're getting the proper, *complete* care that they deserve.

CHAPTER SEVEN

CHIROPRACTIC CARE: THE FIRST OF THE FIVE FACTORS OF HEALTH

The chiropractic approach to disease—and health

The chiropractor approaches disease as a disruption of the "flow of innate," which is causing not only the disease but the symptoms themselves. We address the spine to remove that disruption to allow the innate to flow. In essence, chiropractic does not cure anything; the human body cures itself with our help.

The body has the innate intelligence to heal naturally, though sometimes it needs adjusting to help it along. For example, when we get a cut, our body naturally heals. First it stops the bleeding by coagulating the blood at the area of compromise (the cut); the body automatically knows to send platelets there. Then, new skin and scar tissue is formed, promoting new cell growth. And it all happens exactly where it needs to happen! After all, your body doesn't attempt to heal the cut on your finger by sending new skin to grow on your toe. Sending blood to the "wrong" place by mistake, causing platelets to develop, could ultimately cause a stroke or clog arteries. But the body knows exactly what to do and how to do it. It knows *innately*—intelligently—where the healing needs to take place.

What chiropractic does is allow this innate process to work as flawlessly as it was meant to.

(Note: Again, and you will hear me say this many times during the course of this book: There will always be situations where drastic measures are required. In the case of a heart attack, for example, it doesn't really matter what has caused the heart attack at the moment when the individual lands in the emergency room. There are always going to be situations, given the way we lives our lives, when critical interference will be required to correct an immediate problem. But it remains my belief that medication should only be used in extremely acute cases, and most dire circumstances can be avoided given the right approach to maintaining good health.)

Unfortunately, most of the time, even after the signal (the heart attack, for example) that something is drastically wrong, as soon as the acute situation has passed, we drop the ball. There is little substantive follow-up for the person who's experienced an attack of some kind, little—or no—follow-up to address his or her body's extreme imbalances with anything other than pills (and perhaps a few suggestions for changing dietary habits, etc).

The patient is basically abandoned when there is an abundance that could be offered in terms of chiropractic, acupuncture, massage therapy, and so much more, any or all of which could help that patient improve his or her condition, often significantly. However, the time for a more health-oriented approach to maintain a balanced system is not only *after* the extreme situation, but long before your system has reached the point of extreme crisis.

Recently, there are people who scoff at the idea of inner healing in the practice of health care; in reality, this approach, now aptly called "holistic," was practiced for years without the label attached. If you're anywhere over the age of twenty-five, you probably remember when most Western doctors treated patients with a 'whole-istic' approach, since they were generalists prior to the age of specializing. Pediatricians are actually still generalists to some lesser degree, but after we get to a certain age, it's off to the specialists for just about anything that needs addressing.

There's nothing wrong with seeing someone who specializes in the area you need to address, but whenever you address the micro, the macro can get lost in the process. Holistic medicine attempts to put the big picture back in healthcare. If you've never tried it, you'll be amazed how good it feels to go to a doctor (of chiropractic, acupuncture, etc.) who wants to find out all about *you*, about your life, and your concerns—before trying to uncover the true nature of the symptoms behind those concerns.

The history of chiropractic

The roots of chiropractic care can be traced all the way back to the beginning of recorded time. Writings from China and Greece from as early as 2700 and 1500 BC mention spinal manipulation and the maneuvering of the lower extremities to ease low back pain and achieve health.

The actual profession of chiropractic—as a distinct form of health care—dates back to 1895. As Terry Rondberg noted in his article "Chiropractic First (*Chiropractic Journal, 1996*), Hypocrates himself even endorsed the profession. Hypocrates, a great physician, was a proponent of spinal manipulation . He believed that nature was truly our greatest healer, and that the doctor's only job was to clear away anything that prevented the body from healing itself. He advised us to "get knowledge" of the spine as it is the root cause of many illnesses.

Through the years, people have known that manipulation of the spine helps achieve health, but specific evidence suggesting that specific manipulations at specific points would accomplish healing was still lacking. Only "gross manipulation" (to be discussed below) was practiced until Daniel David Palmer, or D.D. Palmer, discovered what was called the "specific adjustment" in the U.S. in 1895. Born in Canada in 1845, it was Palmer who developed the philosophy of chiropractic that forms the foundation for the profession as it exists today.

When Palmer came to the U.S., he met Harvey Lillard, a janitor who had been deaf for seventeen years. Palmer's subsequent adjustment of Lillard's spine restored his hearing. When Palmer moved to Davenport, Iowa, in 1895, he became familiar with the work of a man named Paul Caster, a magnetic healer. Magnetic healers had been an ongoing phenomenon in America's heartland since the late 1860s and Palmer immediately began studies with Caster. In 1897, Palmer began the Palmer School of Chiropractic, which has continued to be one of the most prominent chiropractic colleges in the nation. It has been said that an early patient of Palmer's, the Reverend Samuel Weed, suggested the name of the profession from the Greek *praxis* (practice) and *cheir* (practice by hand) [*The Chiropractic Profession*, David Chapman-Smith, NCMIC Group, 2007].

Palmer was appreciated for being well read in the medical journals of his time and was up to date with in-depth knowledge of global developments regarding anatomy and physiology. Yet, even years after Lillard's hearing was restored, Palmer was still being vilified by the news media (and the medical community), who persisted in calling him a charlatan. When the medical establishment conspired—and actually succeeded—in having him jailed for practicing medicine without a license, Palmer was sentenced to one hundred and five days and was required to pay a $350 fine.

Way ahead of his time, D.D. Palmer continued to defend himself against the doctors' attacks by presenting arguments against the medical procedures of vaccination and surgery. He also cautioned against introducing medicine into the body, saying it was often unnecessary and even harmful. Palmer fathered a son, B.J., in 1881, who was as enthusiastic about chiropractic as his father and continued D.D.'s work after his death in 1913. B.J. Palmer has been credited for developing chiropractic into a clearly defined and unique healthcare system and was instrumental in chiropractic's ultimate recognition as a licensed profession. Chiropractic doctors continued to gain legal recognition across the US throughout the twentieth century.

In the report *Chiropractic in New Zealand* (published in 1979), the authors strongly supported the efficacy of chiropractic care and elicited medical cooperation in conjunction with it. In 1993, the *Manga* study, published in Canada, investigated the cost effectiveness of chiropractic care. The results concluded that chiropractic care "would save hundreds of millions of dollars annually" in disability and health care costs.

The first state in the U.S. to recognize and license the practice of chiropractic was Minnesota in 1905; Louisiana was the last in 1974. At the current time, doctors of chiropractic normally complete four years at an accredited college of chiropractic, and over 500 hours are devoted to studying adjustive techniques and spinal analysis. Doctors of chiropractic pass a national board examination as well as all exams required by the state in which the individual wishes to practice. The chiropractor must meet all state licensing requirements in order to become a Doctor of Chiropractic.

Against all odds: The Wilk case

Although chiropractic care was licensed as early as 1905, as a profession it continued to suffer from criticism from many sources, particularly the medical establishment. It wasn't until the landmark case of *Wilk vs. the American Medical Association* that history changed for the profession of chiropractic everywhere.

Until 1974, the AMA's established committee on quackery was still openly challenging what it considered to be many unscientific forms of healing, including chiropractic, although some believe this committee was established to undermine chiropractic specifically. Prior to the early 1980s, Principle 3 of the AMA Principles of Medical Ethics stated that "a physician should practice a method of healing founded on a scientific basis" and that he should not "professionally associate with anyone who violates this principle." Until 1983, the AMA still held that it was unethical for medical doctors to associate with "unscientific practitioners," and labeled chiropractic nothing more than an "unscientific cult" (*Wilk v. American Medical Ass'n*, 735 F.2d 217, 7th Cir. 1983).

In 1976, however, Chester Wilk and three other chiropractors sued the AMA, several nationwide healthcare associations, and several physicians for violations of Sections 1 and 2 of the Sherman Antitrust Act (the first United States government action to limit cartels and monopolies, and the oldest of all federal U.S. antitrust laws). In 1980, during a major revision of ethical rules (while the *Wilk* litigation was in progress), the AMA replaced Principle 3, stating that a physician "shall be free to choose whom to serve, with whom to associate, and the environment in which to provide medical services."

The plaintiffs lost at the first trial in 1981, then obtained a new trial on appeal in 1983 because of improper jury instructions and admission of irrelevant and prejudicial evidence (*Wilk v. American Medical Ass'n*, 735 F.2d 217, 7th Cir. 1983).

On September 25, 1987, Judge Getzendanner, the Federal Appeals Court judge on this case, issued her opinion that the AMA had violated only Section 1 of the Sherman Act, and was guilty of illegal conspiracy of systematic long-term wrongdoing and intent to destroy a licensed profession based on an extensive misinformation campaign portraying chiropractic as unscientific, cultist and being incompatible with modern medical practice (*Wilk v. American Medical Ass'n*, 671 F. Supp. 1465, N.D. Ill. 1987).

Getzendanner subsequently issued a permanent injunction against the AMA to prevent this kind of future behavior, indicating tactics the AMA used, including suppressing research favorable to chiropractic, undermining chiropractic education, and using new ethical rulings to prevent cooperation between medical doctors and chiropractors in education. The Court gave judgment against the AMA, involving a multimillion-dollar award of costs and a permanent injunction or restraining order to keep them from maligning chiropractic.

Further, terms were established to enjoin the AMA and anyone associated with it from restricting anyone from associating with chiropractors (*Wilk et al vs. American Medical Association et al.*, U.S. Federal Court Northern District of Illinois, Eastern Division #76C3777; Getzendanner, J., Judgment dated August 27, 1987).

The Court further stood with Wilk's side when it directed that the injunction be sent to all AMA members and that the AMA would be required to publish the injunction in its medical journal. With these acts, there was an immediate and significant increase in chiropractic practice, education and research. Whereas prior to this case, medical doctors were fearful of sending patients to chiropractors for care because they were in jeopardy of losing their hospital privileges (and/or being shunned by the AMA), these same doctors became increasingly likely to refer patients to chiropractors and to begin working in partnership with them.

As a case in point, in a recent article in a publication called *Consumer Reports On Health*, the topic was about alternative treatments of low back pain, and the medical doctors interviewed recognized chiropractic as a viable form of healthcare.

As thrilled as I am with the progress we've made in this direction, I still need to ask, "What's really changed?" Chiropractic is still the same practice it was twenty years ago (albeit an always improving one). Therefore, we can assume that the only thing that has really changed is a shift in thought on the part of the medical establishment. And we can only hope that these collaborative efforts will continue and increase as time goes on.

What is chiropractic?

Since 1974 and the *Wilk* decision, chiropractic care has been growing by leaps and bounds; in fact, chiropractic is the fastest growing and most widely accepted "alternative" form of healthcare today. By the time my children are adults, it is both my hope and expectation that chiropractic will be considered an integral part of mainstream healthcare.

Chiropractic is best described by the quote from Thomas Edison: "The doctor of the future will give no medicine, but will interest his patients in the care of the human frame, in diet, and in the cause and prevention of disease." I believe this statement shows wisdom of incredible foresight, second to none, on a holistic scale because it realizes the fact that the brain is the master controller of the entire body: it tells the heart when to beat, the body to shiver on a cold day, the eyelids to wink.

Every single physiological event that takes place—every movement, thought or sensation—is commanded by the brain. The brain sends its messages telling the body what to do, when to do it, and how to do it down through the spinal cord by way of electrical impulses. The spinal cord acts as a kind of conveyor for all that information to be processed. Fortunately, our spinal cords are protected by a series of bones called vertebrae, or the spine.

How important is the spine to our ability to function? Immeasurable. Consider the fact that the brain and spinal cord are the first two structures to form in an embryo, requiring the nine months of a pregnancy to fully form and then function properly, and without which we could not survive.

The vertebrae move very freely because they're separated by disks. One reason for these disks is to allow enough space for the spinal nerves to exit; the separation gives rise to the IVF, or intervertebral foramen, the hole through which the nerve exits. Occasionally, the vertebral motion segment no longer functions properly, usually due to a vertebra being misaligned, and results in local inflammation around the area of the problem. This inflammation causes a slight pressure on the nerve root called a subluxation.

Vertebral subluxation

You may have also heard the term "vertebral subluxation" if you've experienced certain back symptoms and have been to a chiropractor. In essence, the subluxation is a misalignment that causes abnormal function of the vertebra and the disk. The subsequent abnormal wear and tear causes local inflammation of the surrounding soft tissues (muscles, ligaments and tendons)—and where we have inflammation, we usually have fluid. It's this inflammation that puts pressure on the nerve.

Since our brain uses these nerves (electrical pathways) to send signals to the rest of our body that control and coordinate every single thing our body does, this pressure presents a problem. The energy that flows through us via these electrical pathways is referred to as the *life force*; this is also what chiropractors refer to as our *innate intelligence*. Any time we adjust a patient, we think of it in terms of releasing the power of the innate to start the pathways flowing again in order to restore balance and harmony.

When pressure is placed on the spinal nerve, the body is not in balance. Restoring function through chiropractic adjustment is what causes the inflammation and irritated tissues to normalize. When pressure is removed from the nerve, its function is restored. When the signal travels from the brain to its destination without any interference, our body is in balance.

DIS-EASE PROCESS:
Subluxation (cause) ➡ Pinched nerve (effect) ➡
Damage (usually not noticed) ➡ Symptom
(last thing to present, usually after the damage
has been done)

Why chiropractic?

Although some people don't respond to chiropractic care, the vast majority does. In fact, ninety-two percent of all chiropractic patients respond favorably to the satisfaction of both doctor and patient. So why don't more people explore the benefits of chiropractic care?

There are a number of reasons why chiropractic remains somewhat of a well-kept secret. One is that people simply do not understand what it is and how it works. One of my patients, an athlete and regular triathlon participant, recently shed some light on this conundrum for me.

Holly first came to me for bursitis in her hip that was keeping her from her athletic pursuits due to pain. (Her problem has subsided, but Holly still comes to see me regularly for prophylactic treatments, or, as she says, "just to stay aligned and adjusted.") She sends lots of people to my practice for help, many of whom are athletes like her whose lives have been significantly hindered due to pain of some kind. I asked Holly what she tells people so that they feel inspired to try chiropractic for the first time. This is what she said:

"I tell them pain means something has got to be out of alignment that has to be fixed. I tell them that people don't understand that chiropractic is not just about the spine, even though it starts there! It's about so much more than that. And then I tell them about my own experience and my son's experience. Once I do that, they want to come because they want to get better. They need to try something new, and they decide they want to try chiropractic."

Interview with Holly Tripp

Holly is a 45-year-old woman who runs Ironman triathlons and takes phenomenal care of her body. She runs the spin classes my wife takes and exercise classes at a local gym. Holly has a wide knowledge of many aspects of fitness.

DR. PATON: *Holly, can you tell us what made you come in the first place and why you keep coming?*

HT: The first reason I came was because my hip was hurting and it never stopped hurting. I had very bad bursitis in my right hip. I had to stop marathoning because of it. I couldn't stand it. When I came in, you took x-rays and showed me how my whole back was out of alignment, that my hips were uneven and that's where the problem was. I don't believe in taking pills or doing surgery and wanted to try a different way. And you got my back straightened out. My hip pain is totally gone. It doesn't hurt me to run whatsoever. And every time I have any little problem, you put me back in alignment and the problem is gone.

DR. PATON: *What would you tell someone who doesn't know anything about chiropractic, someone who might exercise regularly but has never seen a chiropractor?*

HT: I always tell people who have trouble, "Just go and give it a try. It's certainly not going to be a bad thing and you never know—it may take care of the problem." Knees, hips…I send everybody to you and they always come out happy. They tell me, "Everything's adjusted; he put everything back where it's supposed to go. The pain is gone."

DR. PATON: *Another patient told me recently that when people ask her what I do for her, she can't explain it. And I realize now it's hard for the layperson to tell people about chiropractic. But you do such a good job of it. You refer so many patients in. How do you do it? How do you explain it to them?*

HT: I think usually it's just telling them what I've been through, telling them that it worked for me and about other people you've helped.

You remember the guy doing marathons who fell down with pain? He fell down after eight miles and we had to get him with a car. I talked him into coming in to see you and give it a try. I told him I *knew* you could change it. Well, he did the marathon about three weeks later. It was a miracle.

I tell people to try it because it's holistic and healthy. Why go to drugs and surgery or anything else if you don't have to?

DR. PATON: *You don't go into a detailed discussion on the mechanics of how it works?*

HT: No, I just tell them something's got to be out of alignment and it has to be fixed.

As far as my kids go, my older son won't go to anyone else—just you—and he's had a lot of broken bones. For example, he broke his ribs in a soccer injury. He was terribly constipated for 4 days post injury. After your exam, you found that as a result of the soccer inury, besides two broken ribs, he had a vertebra misaligned that was related to his intestines. He couldn't move his bowels for days until you started adjusting him. He was in more pain from his gastric track than his ribs. Just keeping him in alignment and helping him heal has provided so much relief for him.

But people don't understand that—they think it's just your spine...I tell them chiropractic is for your whole body!

I am grateful for Holly's help because I have floundered for ways to share the benefits of chiropractic with people who may be less than enthusiastic. I know there are lots of people who simply fear the unknown, or those who would rather trust in the physicians they know or in the pills they can take. I can understand their reticence in trying something new, especially in light of the fact that chiropractic often seems "less" than a quick fix, although it can have immediate positive results and certainly be considered a long-term cure in many instances.

Patience has been said to be a virtue, and never is that truer than when working with chiropractic care. These days, when popping pills for immediate gratification is often the preferred course of action, this kind of treatment can be a tough concept for some people to embrace. But when one treats with chiropractic responsibly and with the patient's best interests and health in mind, effective treatment must run its course.

As I indicated, 92% of all patients of chiropractic respond favorably, and I myself have experienced an incredibly high rate of success—*when my patients commit to the specified treatment course and regimen.* Visits usually decrease over time, of course, but initially the patient has to be willing to commit to the *full course of treatment to experience the desired results.*

As I write this book (in 2008), the average chiropractic treatment plan is anywhere from $700 to $1200. Once most patients consider that time alone has not improved their symptoms prior to coming in to see me, or how they have been existing on painkillers and muscle relaxants without improvement, or how much their symptoms are actually worsening and could make it necessary for them to have surgery (which could easily run into sixty to one hundred thousand dollars), they often decide they want to try a course of chiropractic first!

Conceptually, we can think of it the way we think of so many other options and opportunities. If you don't take care of a cavity, it can easily turn into a root canal—or you could ultimately lose the tooth altogether. The goal of chiropractic is to restore balance in the body and put you back on a general course of good health as efficiently and effectively as possible—in other words, to improve your quality of life for the long run.

How long does treatment last?

In my office, twenty-four to twenty-eight treatments is the average course to successfully treat a misalignment of the spine. (Remember, the spine is where the trouble is often located, but not necessarily where the pain is felt.) However, that merely represents the treatment for the typical or average patient in my office. That number of treatments is tailored to each patient and may increase or decrease, depending on the severity of the spinal misalignment, level of arthritic degeneration, or the type of technique that the chiropractor utilizes.

Because the treatment plan is an important part of whether or not the treatment will be successful, those who don't follow their doctor's instructions and quit the treatment prematurely can often be heard to disparage chiropractic, insisting that it did not do what was originally promised. I'd love to see a patient before a surgery tell the orthopedic surgeon, "Even though you told me this surgery will take 2 hours, I want you to close me up in 15 minutes and I'll go see if it'll work or not." Then, when it doesn't work, would they go around saying negative things about the surgeon? It simply wouldn't happen.

Chiropractic can be compared to orthodontic work. It takes at least a year of treatments to reset a mouth full of misaligned teeth, and then, after that, a retainer to keep the realigned teeth in place so that the treatment will hold. Getting on board with the treatment means staying with the program until the whole course has been run. The same is true for a chiropractic treatment plan, in which the patient and the problem need to be guided over time to have the changes last. When one adheres to the program, chiropractic can provide a total recovery, the same way orthodontic can provide a whole new smile.

Keep in mind that chiropractic does not mask the pain the way a pill does. We all know, though we may like to think otherwise, that not everything responds to a pill or potion, and that's where chiropractic comes in. Chiropractic treats the cause of the problem so pills become a thing of the past.

Putting your trust in your chiropractic provider not only means getting better, but *getting better faster—and more naturally.*

Happy patients make a happy chiropractor

One reason I find it so satisfying to be a chiropractor is because I see so many happy faces. There is a reason so many of my patients are happy when they come into my office: their general sense of well-being.

Although these people initially came to see me with the same kinds of problems you may have—stress, physical disabilities, pain, etc.—they are now feeling so good that they are able to deal with the curve balls that life eventually tosses to us all.

The curve ball

One day your boss comes over and says, "This project needs to be completed two days earlier than expected, so I need it on my desk by tomorrow afternoon." "No problem, boss," you say, but as you head back to your office, you feel the onset of your first headache of the week. The tightness is already creeping into your neck and shoulders as you think about how you might miss your daughter's soccer game and that it's your wife's birthday and, if you don't hurry, you might not have time to buy her a present.

Question: Which person would you rather be? (1) The person who has neck and shoulder tightness, headaches, and back pain; has suffered from similar symptoms in the past; and who worries now how, given his pain and discomfort, he will ever get the job done on time; (2) the person with the same symptoms who takes muscle relaxants (that often make him feel as if he's in a fog and make it even harder to get the job done) and anti-inflammatories (that caused stomach ulcers to erupt in the past); or (3) the person who gets occasional but regular chiropractic adjustments so that even though he feels understandably annoyed with his boss, he remains clear, awake, pain-free, and ready to take on the challenge?

For me—and for most chiropractic patients—it's a no-brainer. Yet many of the people reading this book struggle with the idea that something as relatively "simple" as a chiropractic adjustment could have such a resoundingly positive effect.

They struggle because they've heard that chiropractic is something to be afraid of or they've rejected it out of hand as a possible alternative—even though the only thing they may know about the subject might be from a source who has probably never experienced chiropractic treatment before!

What really happens in the chiropractic office

Later in this book, you'll read about a number of patients who came to my office virtually, if not literally, kicking and screaming. They came because they had nowhere else to turn, because their mothers made them promise, or they were bringing someone else to see me. You'll read their own descriptions of how their disbelief about chiropractic turned to belief and how they now share their stories so that other people won't have to live through the pain the way they did.

That's why most of my patients are referred to me.

I don't have to advertise because my patients constantly tell people they know to give chiropractic a chance. This philosophy allows me to use the money I would otherwise spend on advertising to philanthropically donate to good causes and to the community, and that's a beautiful thing to be able to do for humanity. Patient referrals like these happen when—and because—patients get better.

A patient referral will often mean that the new patient knows at least one other person who has benefited from chiropractic care. That makes it a bit easier when it comes to offsetting any apprehension the patient might have because he/she has already talked to a friend, colleague or family member who helped alleviate their fears. They are aware of the basics of chiropractic treatment and are eager to get started. They have decided that the wild rumors that have dogged chiropractic (at least in the past) are not worth consideration.

When a patient comes for the first visit, h/she fills out paperwork related to health and HIPPA guidelines (for patient protection), then meets with me for a consultation. During that time, I ask specific questions regarding the chief complaint and create in my mind what's called a differential diagnosis from a whole list of possibilities. As I ask more and more questions regarding the patient's chief complaint, I cross out possibilities, narrowing the list.

After the consult, which includes discussion of any other health issues the patient wants to talk about, we go into the exam room, where we normally take pictures of the spine. X-rays provide something very much akin to a roadmap when driving to a previously unknown destination, because you can only do so much by feeling the musculature, vertebra, etc. For example, you wouldn't want to misinterpret a genetic abnormality by treating it as a new injury of some kind. (Occasionally, a patient will tell me he's never had x-rays performed although he's been adjusted for years. My typical response is that x-rays are a technological advancement with tremendous benefits, depending on the situation and the patient's complaints.)

More on the subject of x-rays

X-rays are often necessary to understand the complete picture of any patient's condition prior to treatment. Naturally, chiropractors try to avoid any undue x-rays, but you should try to appreciate the practitioner's suggestions for treatment in this regard.

When I had my x-ray machine installed, I was concerned about the radiation exposure and made it my business to pay an x-ray physicist to guide me on how much lead I would need in the office walls to protect myself and everyone in, and around, my office. The physicist told me that an airline pilot absorbs more x-radiation from a single transcontinental flight than one x-ray puts out from my machine.

To a medical doctor, x-rays are, in fact, useless in most cases of low back pain. Their treatment—"wait to see what happens and start drug therapy"—is not contingent upon the x-rays and what they show. To a medical doctor, an x-ray is "normal" if there's no fracture or no tumor. If they see arthritis, the treatment will focus on that arthritis—not on its cause, which is usually due to some kind of misalignment and, hence, an imbalance. They will treat it with anti-inflammatories and painkillers.

On occasion, when no fracture, tumor or arthritis is discovered on an x-ray, the radiology report reads: "No anomalies, normal finding." The patient will often arrive at my office and say, "My doctor told me that everything is fine but I'm not making this pain up!" Sometimes they're very emotional because they were offended when their doctor recommended that they go on antidepressants.

When I take my own x-rays, I'm baffled when I see how misaligned these same patients' spines are. I wonder why the initial x-ray report suggested "normal findings" because, although there might not have been any tumor or fracture, it was far from normal! It was clear to see the spinal misalignments that were causing the pinched nerves (which were thus causing the excruciating pain).

Rapport

As a chiropractor, I try to create an immediate rapport with a patient, to create an atmosphere of trust, and I do this quietly and with focus. I focus my energies on that patient like an eagle; I really think hard about that patient, connect with him, let him know he won't be treated like anyone else, and that he'll be treated with care and attention.

I may ask a few personal questions, but largely the focus is on trying to let the patient feel the positive energy—because that's where the first stage of healing begins. Once patients know they are in the right place, the *qi* (the body's life force) will start to flow and the healing can begin—even before I have laid a hand on them.

There's one thing I feel I must mention here. There are all sorts of healthcare providers, all sorts of healthcare provider offices, and all sorts of staff. Where an office is chaotic, dirty or disorganized, or where the provider talks about how he couldn't go boating or to his golf game, I don't believe the healing can ever even begin.

I take great pride in the fact that in my office, patients who come in with pain can expect an exam and a *relief treatment* on the first day. A "relief treatment" compares to a regular treatment in that I haven't had time to review any x-rays yet. Relief treatment is a gentle stretch just like *qi gong*, the ancient form of treatment where the practitioner doesn't touch the patient, but rather treats by the transfer of energy from his hand directly to the patient.

Of course, a majority of my patients come to my office for stiff necks or low back spasms, and most of them are on some type of over-the-counter or prescription medication. When I ask them if the medication is working, 99% answer, "No." Otherwise, I would have to assume that they were happy with their mode of treatment and would not have found their way to my office.

In most cases, after a few adjustments, their pain recedes, as do the spasms. After a few more adjustments, the spine starts to stabilize, and at that point the pain will likely disappear for good because the normal motion has been slowly restored to the vertebral motion segment, which took the pressure off the nerve that was causing the pain.

Sometimes the affected or irritated nerve goes to the neck, sometimes to the low back, and other times to other areas, such as around the intestines, stomach, or sinuses. A patient once came to my office from the gym next door. She wanted to be adjusted for several reasons: she had neck pain and was concerned that she would be feeling uncomfortable for her wedding, which was taking place in two weeks' time; she had a small hump forming on the back of her lower neck (called Dowager's Hump) and was very self-conscious about it; and she had low back pain that would come and go.

I performed a history and exam and took x-rays on this young woman's first visit. I went over her x-rays with her on the second visit and explained what we needed to do. I also asked her if she had any problems with IBS (Irritable Bowel Syndrome). Her eyes got wide and she said, "Yes! How did you know that?" I told her I could see it in her spine from the first lumbar vertebra's being out of alignment; that vertebra contains the nerve that innervates the intestines. She informed me that during her childhood, she'd experienced many problems with IBS. She also told me that she was hesitant to go out sometimes because she thought she'd need to go to the bathroom.

Her mother worked at one of the larger, well known cancer hospitals in the area. Consequently, she had her daughter tested by very renowned doctors who put her on several different medications with several side effects. After all the testing was complete, my patient was told there was "nothing wrong" and that she needed to live with her symptoms.

After the first couple of adjustments in my office, her neck began feeling better; after a few more, she said that her friends noticed the hump was decreasing. She was no longer self-conscious about wearing her wedding dress. After another couple of treatments, her IBS stopped.

The chiropractic body detective

It may sound a little hokey but when I get a new patient, I (along with many chiropractors) like to think that I look at his or her body with the eyes of a detective—a body detective.

Pain in a joint, for example, doesn't necessarily mean that the joint needs to be manipulated or adjusted. Chiropractic's first goal is to identify the real cause of the patient's symptoms, then find a way to alleviate those symptoms—not to chase the symptoms with mitigating drugs.

I often give this example to patients, athletic trainers, and medical doctors: If you put your arm over the back of a chair and press hard enough in the arm pit area, your hand will go numb. There are two schools of thought about how to address the numbness in the hand. One, inject the hand with some kind of anti-inflammatory to calm down the nerve; or, two, take the pressure off the nerve where it's being pinched—under the arm.

That's just one good example of how medical providers differ in approach from chiropractors, who make it their life's work to attempt to find and correct the cause of the symptoms.

The focus is on the spine

Chiropractors' first and foremost goal—what they are trained to do—is to adjust the spine to restore its normal function. In aligning the spine correctly, pressure can be taken off the nerves, which then allows your body to express its full potential—without pain.

Chiropractic is not only for emergency or pain-related situations. It can also be used effectively for ongoing wellness care, to help keep you healthy and balanced in times of less stress so that you are better prepared for the times that get tough.

I have to admit that it can be frustrating for me *and* for the patients whom I treat when they tell me about their friends and family members who have such pain in their bodies but refuse to try chiropractic. My patients try and try to get these people—who are in pain with "bad backs" and "old sports injuries"—to a chiropractor's office to help them with all kinds of symptoms. Because they have experienced the "miracle" of chiropractic, they want their loved ones to experience the benefits, too.

And miracles happen all the time. Children come in with ear infections and, a few treatments later, are completely without infection and pain; patients come in with Irritable Bowel Syndrome and, after a series of treatments, experience totally normal digestive patterns; others come in with migraine headaches that improve with every single treatment until they are often completely migraine-free.

I'd be willing to bet that many of you reading this right now are thinking, "Come on, you can't treat those conditions. Chiropractors just 'pop the spine.'" And yes, it's true—we *do* adjust the spine. But as you read this book, you will realize why chiropractic is so effective in helping so many conditions, and how chiropractic is much bigger than relieving the neck and back pain for which it's known.

The past, the present and the future

Two high school students recently approached me with a request to help them with their research for their yearlong class project. Their task was to locate a professional in an occupation that interested them, meet with the professional throughout the year, and learn all they could about the occupation in preparation for possibly considering a career in that field.

I was very flattered to find out that they wanted to meet with me, and last night we had our first meeting. As we started to discuss their project, the first thing they shared with me was the resistance they'd encountered when they made the decision to make their topic/occupation the field of chiropractic. I was stunned to find out that in their high school, there are still people who, although they've never been to a chiropractor, feel free to insist that chiropractic is some kind of mystical medicine, something less than legitimate.

Some typical comments, by adults and teens alike, directed at these students were: "Oh, you want to be a *chiropractor*? They don't do anything for anybody;" "How do you know you want to be a chiropractor? My mother went to one once and it didn't help at all;" "Oh…*chiropractors*. Well, I guess that's okay." Unfortunately, this is a representative sample of what the American public has been led to believe about chiropractic.

Both of these students were patients of mine already. The young woman had suffered from constant headaches until she got adjusted; she had an obvious zeal for chiropractic. Lisa told me that when her Mom was young, she was a cheerleader and gymnast and, as a result, now suffers from chronic back pain. Lisa's Mom told her how she wishes she'd seen a chiropractor herself. However, seeing her daughter suffer was enough to try chiropractic because she didn't want Lisa on prescription drugs to treat her symptoms. Lisa confirmed at this point that her headaches were gone and she was taking no medications whatsoever.

Tom, the young man, said, "I suffered a lot with allergies and other things. Now I sleep a lot better." Lisa and Tom both told me that they met with responses of disbelief when they shared their own stories of how they'd been helped with chiropractic, that chiropractic wasn't simply for neck and back pain, and that they were determined to become chiropractors themselves. I was impressed at how these two were making up their own minds and not letting other peoples' opinions sway their desire and drive.

I congratulated these students on their tenaciousness and ability to see beyond the attitudes of some people, which keep them missing out on true, good healthcare. Level of education, position or intelligence doesn't always mean "smart" because there is no substitute for finding a valid source of information. I also reminded them that experiencing the benefits of chiropractic is ultimately the only answer people need.

Balancing the body through chiropractic care

We have to face the reality that drug companies will not be relinquishing their hold on us any time soon. There are also going to be situations where drugs play an important role in our survival. With that said, chiropractic can provide a way to offset the need for drugs for many people.

The premise of chiropractic care is that by balancing the body and keeping it aligned, it will stay healthy. There are four other factors (which will be discussed in later chapters) that contribute to that balancing process. When one or more of those factors is lacking, you can't have overall maximized health. For example, if a person were to get adjusted every day, but also subsisted on junk food twice a day and avoided exercise, adjusting would not be enough to keep him balanced and healthy. Chiropractic emphasizes that even if such a person becomes obese and eventually requires medicine for hypertension (high blood pressure), that approach should be only temporary until the patient can effectively change his lifestyle.

What is interesting is that so many people are willing to stay on medications virtually forever but are worried about becoming "addicted" to chiropractic care! One patient actually told me, "I wouldn't go to a chiropractor because I heard that once you go one time, you get addicted and have to go forever." I have to presume they are talking about what we in the profession call "maintenance" care. In that case, patients generally see me only as they feel necessary, and once every few months to stay healthy and happy is average.

What else do chiropractors do?

A large part of any initial course of chiropractic treatment is the report of findings. This is where I explain the process of chiropractic care and the nature of the patient's problem, and set them up on a care plan.

When they finally arrive at my doorstep, many of my patients are almost desperate to find some help for their problems. At this point, they trust they need help, but are often admittedly—and with good reason—skeptical about whether they will get the help they need. After all, they've been to medical doctors of all kinds, have taken many different medications, have experienced many negative side effects, and are often at their wit's end.

Often, these are people who never gave chiropractic a thought as a viable treatment option in the past, but due to their continued pain and/or continued lack of progress, are willing to try just about anything.

Of course, it is true that chiropractic cannot fix everything. There have been many occasions when I have had to refer patients out to medical doctors (cardiologists, orthopedic surgeons, neurologists, and primary care physicians) to meet their needs. I truly believe, for example, that everyone should get regular yearly medical exams—but if you practice the five factors of health, you will most likely pass them with flying colors.

However, patients who live less than optimum lifestyles may have warning signs of blockages in their arteries or other indicators for concern. When people don't practice the five factors of health, they are at extreme risk for medical problems as they get older. When I see a woman who is overweight, doesn't exercise, smokes, drinks and takes birth control, I perform extra tests because she is at a much higher risk of suffering a stroke sooner or later, whether from the side effects of prescription medication or lifestyle choices. Going to a cardiologist for a stress test and ultrasound to rule out potentially deadly conditions can be critically necessary for such patients.

Medicine and chiropractic *can* work well together—and help many people live healthier lives. Using chiropractic in no way diminishes the need for medicine either, since: (1) we will always have acute injuries such as broken bones, lacerations, brain injuries, etc, that require immediate medical intervention, and (2) we will always have unhealthy people who choose not to practice the five factors of health.

Of these five factors, I chose to address chiropractic care first because it helps to balance the body and allow it to practice its innate intelligence. This ability will assist in carrying out the other four factors as well.

CHAPTER EIGHT

THE MECHANICS OF CHIROPRACTIC CARE

Connecting the spine and the nerves

Since chiropractic treatment is the first of the five factors for optimum health, it's important to understand how it can help you lead a healthier overall life. Below is a list that correlates spinal vertebrae with the functions the nerves perform. For example, adjusting the T12/L1 area can help the symptoms of IBS or Irritable Bowel Syndrome.

(see chart page 155)

- C1: Headaches, hypertension, dizziness (thought to be the most powerful adjustment in the human body)
- C2: Sinus trouble, allergies
- C3: Neuralgia
- C4/C5: Throat conditions, pain or numbness in shoulders
- C6: Tonsillitis, stiff neck, pain or numbness in thumb and index finger
- C7: Thyroid conditions, pain or numbness in middle finger
- T1: Asthma, cough, shortness of breath, pain or numbness in ring and pinky finger
- T2: Functional heart conditions
- T3: Bronchitis, lung congestion
- T4: Gall bladder problems

- T5: Liver conditions
- T6: Stomach trouble, acid reflux
- T7: Pancreatic / diabetic conditions (Type 1 diabetics should NOT stop taking insulin)
- T8: Spleen / lowered resistance
- T9: Allergies, increased stress levels
- T10: Kidneys, chronic tiredness
- T11: Kidneys, also acne / skin conditions
- T12: Gas pains
- L1: Constipation, other digestive disorders / pain or numbness in groin
- L2: Cramping in abdomen / pain or numbness in mid-thigh
- L3: Bladder trouble, painful periods (female) / pain or numbness in lower thigh, above knee
- L4: Sciatica, prostate problems (male) / pain or numbness in inside leg, below knee
- L5: leg cramps / pain or numbness in outside leg, below knee
- S1: Sacroiliac conditions / pain or numbness in back of calf

The back

It is obvious from the list above that chiropractic can go a long way in treating many physical ailments, allowing patients to live better, fuller lives.

However, the area of the body with which chiropractic is most often associated is the back—and it is true that back pain prohibits many people from achieving the things they would like to do, not to mention enjoying everyday activities. So it is here that I would like to discuss how the back functions, how the back (as a system) can cause disturbance in the body overall, and how its manipulation can have profound effect on the body as a whole. I'd also like to address some people's concerns about chiropractic adjustments placing undue stress on the spine.

How the lumbar (lower) spine really works

There is considerable evidence suggesting that the cause of catastrophic lower back pain and injury (disc herniation or disk prolapse) commonly relates to one's posture and body position during lifting, as well as the load one is lifting, the element of muscle fatigue, and other factors.

But everyday back pain occurs more easily and is in fact the second-leading reason for loss of work. In *Lumbosacral Disk Injuries*, author Robert E Windsor, M.D., President and Director, Georgia Pain Physicians, PC; Clinical Associate Professor, Department of Physical Medicine and Rehabilitation, Emory University, provides an estimate of 175.8 million days of restricted activity in the US every year due to back pain, and almost 2.5 million Americans experiencing disabling lower back pain.

Frankly, what this means for you and me is that our spines are not only constantly at risk from heavy lifting, but also from activities we do every single day, often repetitively, due to work, and also during daily situations such as brushing our teeth and leaning over the sink. Sinks and countertops in America are so low, for example, that we don't have to be very tall to have to bend significantly to brush our teeth, wash our faces, etc.—and that puts excessive pressure on the spine.

You may think that something as minor as leaning over the counter to brush your teeth couldn't possibly cause something as catastrophic as a disc prolapse. But it can. A study published in the journal *Spine* indicates that out of the various postures tested, the one most likely to cause the disc to prolapse is bending and twisting. If you're like most people (guys in particular), when you finish brushing your teeth, you bend forward and twist your body to slurp some water out of the faucet. This is probably the most dangerous position in which you place your body all day!

In contrast, when we sleep, the discs don't have to support the weight of our bodies, and thus aren't being compressed. Fluid that normally squeezes out of the disc while we're standing all day eventually seeps back into the disc while we sleep. The discs, in other words, rehydrate themselves overnight.

The same study in *Spine*, however, suggests that discs are even more prone to prolapse when they are "oversaturated" first thing in the morning; after the fluid in the disc re-enters the vertebra as the day goes on, the risk of injury decreases (Lu, Y. Michael, PhD; Hutton, William C., DSc; Gharpuray, Vasanti M., PhD. *Do Bending, Twisting, and Diurnal Fluid Changes in the Disc Affect the Propensity to Prolapse? A Viscoelastic Finite Element Model. Spine*, 21(22) 15 Nov. 1996, pp. 2570-2579).

So, if you're not planning on raising the level of your sink, always remember to bend with your knees and use a cup to rinse. Also try to do a few non-weight-bearing stretches (the ones you do lying down) in bed before you get up and move around. Simply pull one knee to your chest and hold it for 30 seconds, then repeat with the opposite leg. Then pull both legs to your chest and let the lower body roll side to side while keeping your shoulders flat on the bed. Doing this for only half a minute will ensure a positive benefit to starting your day—and your back—off right.

Disk herniation and disk prolapse explained

Look at the diagram to identify one of the areas called a "motion segment." Each motion segment includes a vertebra up above, a vertebra down below, and a disk between the two; the disk has a jelly-like substance called a nucleus. The nucleus normally stays right in the middle of the disk because the disk has hundreds to thousands of annular fibers that run almost diagonally through it, right to left and left to right, to keep the nucleus in place.

When the vertebra is aligned properly, the fibers are taut; when the vertebra is rotated, the fibers are less tight, which gives that nucleus a chance to migrate. The only way it can migrate during a motion such as bending forward is posteriorly, or towards the back of the body, because of the intense load put on the lumbar spine during this movement.

Typically, just to lean forward, the spine has to exert an effort equal to at least 2000 pounds to lift your body from a bending position to a full standing position. When the vertebrae rotate left or right, the annular fibers aren't as strong because they're no longer taut. This weakness allows the nucleus (the jelly-like material) to migrate. It is during this process that tears occur in the annular fibers.

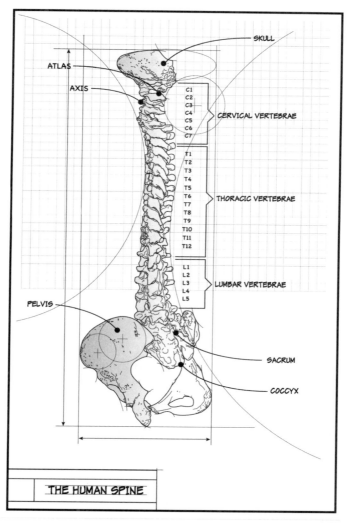

THE HUMAN SPINE

Disk tears (or tears of the annular fibers) can also be caused by dehydration of the disks. As the disks become severely dehydrated, they lose a substantial amount of flexibility. Without flexibility or elasticity, spinal movements can cause the fibers to tear. In these situations, with or without disk tears, it is perfectly safe to be adjusted.

Putting stress on the spine

To show you just how safe a chiropractic treatment is, I will use an example I learned in a post-graduate class called Kinesiology of Sport. The professor, a Ph.D. and an all-American shot putter, talked a lot and in significant detail about the amount of force the spine has to exert during different activities.

One specific activity we looked at was "good mornings," an activity often performed in a gym. In this exercise, weight is suspended on the shoulders, as the person bends forward at the waist. The correct posture is with the spine kept rigid and the knees having a slight bend in them. After bending forward to the point that the chest is almost parallel to the ground, the person comes back up to a standing position. In this class we studied what happened when performing these exercises.

In general, at the maximum movement (when one is bent over the most), the weight used was approximately a "5 rm effort"—in other words, this was the maximum weight the subject could do five times to the point of fatigue. While standing, the angle of the pelvis/lumbar spine was 74.6 degrees. Bent, this angle drops down to a maximum of 19.6 degrees when performing the "good morning" with the chest nearly parallel to the floor. The amount of weight used was very heavy (325 kg) in our example, but the subject was not just any subject—he was a power lifter.

The amount of force his muscles had to exert was astronomical! The spine had to exert 2,963 pounds just to stand upright with the weight on his shoulders. At the point of maximum flexion, at 19.6 degrees, the spine had to exert 8,531 pounds just to hold it in that position. This data was collected in a static (non-moving) position. If we measured the amount of force it took to move the body from the bent-over position to the standing position, the maximum force his muscles would have to exert could reach 17,000 pounds!

So, to give you some perspective, the amount of pressure that a chiropractor uses to administer an adjustment is anywhere from a few ounces to maybe 2-5 pounds per square inch and, with babies, only a few ounces of pressure (far less than is required to pull and twist an infant's head in order to pull him out of the birth canal).

Obviously, adjustments are a far cry less than the 8,531 pounds that the spine can withstand, as illustrated above.

Therefore, there is no doubt that a spinal adjustment is perhaps one of the safest—and beneficial—things you could do to your spine!

The "military neck"

Most people have straight necks, or what's called a *military neck*. In other words, they have lost their neck curves. Sometimes this progresses to a *reversed curve* of the cervical spine, in which the disks wear out prematurely; this is a condition we really need to address.

When the neck has a normal backwards curvature, the majority of the head's weight is dispersed through the joints, the articular pillars. With a straight neck, the disks absorb the majority of the head's weight—the disks weren't meant to take that kind of weight. Their whole purpose is to allow for coupled motion so we have a full range of motion of the neck and also to separate the vertebrae enough to allow each spinal nerve to exit.

When those disks wear out, not only do you lose range of motion, but the spinal nerves get pressure put on them, and sometimes this pressure (called impingement) can get so bad that there's nothing any chiropractor can do. When that happens, there's only one choice: surgery.

In these extreme cases, the disk has fully degenerated to a bone-on-bone state and spurs form which encroach onto the little hole where the nerve comes out. The nerve gets pinched permanently from that bone spur. But that's rare. In the majority of cases, as long as there is joint space there, a chiropractor can work with it. That's why I always say don't jump to surgery!

A chiropractic patient's perspective

Since there is obviously so much that chiropractic care can do to restore the body's balance and alleviate the causes of painful physical symptoms, it is important to hear from someone who has undergone this kind of life-changing treatment. The following story also shows how "back injuries" affect other areas in the body

Brian is a retired Associate Director of Health Services at a state university. He has an extensive knowledge of the healthcare system as well as the greater medical profession, and he is also undergoing chiropractic treatment. What follows is our extensive interview, in which we hear from Brian as both a medical professional and a chiropractic patient.

DR. PATON: *Brian, maybe you could start with an account of what was going on prior to your coming in to receive chiropractic care. Give us an idea of the problems you were experiencing and different modalities and treatments you received and how those treatments came about. I'd also like you to talk at some point about your concerns and fears before coming to a chiropractor, but let's start with your history.*

BRIAN: My back pain started about 2½ years ago. I fell over backwards in the bathroom and hit my back on the edge of the toilet seat. It hurt at the time, but not terribly much, and I thought it was just something that would go away. The pain continued for about a good three months, though, and was worsening.

It happened that I had a doctor of internal medicine who was working for me at the time and whose husband had a pain clinic. Nobody had taken much interest—my own doctor just said it would get better eventually—so I went to the pain clinic and the doctor there obviously suspected something because he immediately ordered an MRI and he wanted it done in a hurry.

So he arranged for the MRI the same day, which I did, and he told me the next day that he wanted me to see a surgeon because he thought that the injury to my back was really serious. He said that if something wasn't done soon, I could lose mainly the nerves necessary for my bladder function and my bowel function. So he contacted "Dr. D." and sent him the MRI and Dr. D. agreed with him that the damage was at L3-4 (I think) and was really dangerous, and he put me into the hospital for an operation within two days.

He explained at the time that there were two injuries and why he wanted to do the upper one first. He said that once he went in there, he and his partner would take a look at the lower, second one and decide if they would do both together or just do the top one.

So I went in and had a laminectomy done on the top one. They looked at the bottom one and decided it wasn't necessarily that dangerous and didn't need to be done right away. Subsequently, I found out that they were hoping that it would just fix itself. To tell you the truth, now, looking back, if I'd known about you at that time, I think it was probably fixable without surgery, but I didn't know and I hadn't thought of chiropractic.

After surgery, they sent me to physiotherapy but the pain continued. I was managing to do the physiotherapy without too much problem but really wasn't getting better. In fact, I was getting worse. So I went back to the pain clinic and he said, "Let's try steroid injections"— which he did. It helped the area of the laminectomy, but didn't touch the lower problem and I was having pretty bad sciatic pain again. But again the only treatment anyone offered me was physiotherapy.

DR. PATON: *I know the British say "physiotherapy"…I believe you mean "physical therapy," where you do exercises and they put the stimulation on you, right?*

BRIAN: Yes. And I was managing but it wasn't fixing the problem. I lifted the weights, rode the bike, did all that, but it wasn't having any permanent effect of any kind. So we did the injections, which didn't help either.

So the pain clinic sent me back to the surgeon who said, "Let's wait and see what happens." Again, I felt that he was hoping that the physiotherapy would fix the problem. At one time I had hopes that it would, too, because I was having an easier and easier time actually doing the physiotherapy but the pain was continuing.

So I went back to the pain clinic again. He did another MRI and CT scan. That was the first time anyone told me that I had scoliosis. He asked me if I was aware that I had "bad scoliosis" and I said no, I wasn't. By this time, the surgeon was saying all they could do was operate on the lower injury and fuse the vertebrae together. And again I didn't know about you or chiropractic or anything else. So I went back for the second surgery and it did help somewhat, at least it got rid of the sciatic pain, but I was still in a lot of pain and

I couldn't figure out why. But that time my insurance company wouldn't pay for more physiotherapy, so it was decided that I would try to do it at home and continue what they'd taught me.

That was when my daughter was visiting you as a chiropractor—I don't think I had known that at the time. I didn't even know she had a problem—and I still don't really know what it is. But she kept telling me that this doctor was really good and why didn't I go see him?

Now, many years ago—probably 35 years ago—I had one treatment of chiropractic. I was living in Canada at the time and a friend of mine had studied chiropractic there. He was fairly fresh out of college. I'd had a minor injury of my shoulder and asked him if he could help. But what it entailed was tremendous gyrations of my body, having to twist my legs and back while he wrapped his arms around my whole body and did all kinds of things…it was painful.

When he worked on my head and jammed it sideways, I thought he was going to break something. However, to be honest, he fixed my shoulder. But it made me very nervous about going to a chiropractor ever again. If it takes that just for a little shoulder injury, I thought, what happens if you really need something done? I don't know whether it was because he'd trained in Canada, or because it was so long ago, but the way that he did chiropractic—and the way *you* do chiropractic—is vastly different.

So, when my daughter came to me and told me to see you, I told her I really had enough pain and really didn't need any more. She said, "Look, I've spoken to him and explained that you've got a fusion." And that was the part that scared me, that if you didn't know what you were doing, you might damage that area even worse and I'd find myself back in surgery. She said, "I have faith in this guy. I don't think he would do anything like that. Besides, all I want him to do is have a look and get his opinion. I'm quite sure if he feels he might damage something or that he might not be able to help, that he'll tell you."

So I came to your office. Now, I've worked in medicine since I was eighteen. As a professional, I'm a clinical chemist and moved from that into management when I was about thirty and I worked in hospitals in three different countries and I have met a lot of doctors and have a pretty good idea of how to sum them up, I think, anyway. And in my estimation, there are a lot more bad ones than good ones. And when I got to your office, I was immediately impressed with the surroundings and with the help…I think you can tell a lot about a doctor from his staff. If they are well-trained, competent, treat the patient well, it gives you a feeling of being comfortable. That probably means the doctor knows what he's doing because he's got a decent staff…

DR. PATON: *I feel the same way and that's why we work so hard on that.*

BRIAN: And it's worth it. They are very helpful, very professional. So from there, I could see when I looked at the x-ray that my back was far worse than I had imagined it to be. I had an idea what scoliosis was but not really, and I hadn't given it that much thought. I was more concerned with what had happened in the areas of the two operations because at the top one there was a definite curve in my back and the bottom one obviously had the fusion.

Now, my father had a back condition. I don't know what it was but I do know he had a curved back by the time he died at about 67. I thought that maybe it was just genetics and nobody could do anything about it. But I thought I'd see what you had to say about it. And then you examined me and showed me the x-ray and what I really appreciated was you said right up front that at 67 years old, you couldn't give me the back of a 17-year-old, but you believed you could help me. Then you said, "I do believe I can help you without hurting you or certainly without any permanent damage. So why don't we give it a try? If you don't like it, you can stop any time," and this seemed reasonable to me.

I was dreading it but, again, I was anticipating the kind of treatment I'd gotten back in Canada. First you had me get on the chair with the rollers but the pain was too much in the area of the first operation.

DR. PATON: *You're referring here to the intersegmental traction table, where you lie down and it rolls up and down your back to loosen the spine, right?*

BRIAN: Yes, and that pain was too much and so the girl stopped the machine immediately and told you. Then I had my first examination where you adjusted me a little. And I thought, that's it? That's what he's going to do? [Laughter]

DR. PATON: [Laughing, too] *A lot of people say that.*

BRIAN: Because I felt nothing. I didn't have to do weird contortions and you weren't forcing and twisting my head… So my daughter and I talked about it when I left and I said, "You know, I agree with you that if nothing else, I don't think this doctor is going to do me any harm. He appears to be fairly optimistic that he can help me. I'm realistic that at my age he can't cure me—that's probably impossible—I'll always have back trouble, but if he can improve what's happening to me, I'll try it."

At that point, I was really starting to deteriorate a bit; it was getting harder to walk, I had to use my cane, my balance was quite bad, and the pain was pretty bad. Nowhere near like it was before the second operation, but still pretty bad. And there are still days where it gets pretty painful, to tell you the truth. But I decided to see if you could really help me. Somehow you engendered my trust. I thought that what you were telling me was probably true and I didn't expect a cure, but I thought if you could improve to make my life less uncomfortable then I would have achieved what I wanted to achieve.

As we worked, your adjustments were so gentle that I wondered if you were really achieving very much. As time went by, it appeared to me that the adjustments were getting a little more pressured. I was able to go back on the table and without a doubt I was feeling better. I was still having quite a few bad days but I was having some good days, too.

And it's continued to where we've reached the stage now whether I honestly don't know if you can make it any better. You might be able to, but I've accepted the fact that I'm old and that my back is in bad shape. But you have greatly improved the quality of my life. I can now walk fairly comfortably around the house all day without any problem. I can go out, that kind of thing.

DR. PATON: *Many people have that pill popper mentality where they want to see it get better overnight and that makes them drop out of treatment before they ever get to see the benefits of chiropractic. But you stuck with it. And I would love to figure out why you did. Because it's frustrating for me when people I believe I can help leave before they get that help. Can you tell me why you trusted us enough to stay?*

BRIAN: Well, it was a combination of factors. I felt comfortable. I felt that you were helping me. And really it was just the professional way you were going about things…you didn't make any promises you couldn't keep.

DR. PATON: *Have you gone back and told your previous physicians about your progress with chiropractic and, if so, what was their reaction?*

BRIAN: My internist said he was very pleased that I'd come to you and that if I'd asked him he would have encouraged me because he has found that a lot of patients get helped with a good chiropractor.

In America, it gets drummed into us at a such an early age—particularly someone like myself, who's been in medicine—that chiropractic is not that wonderful, that chiropractors don't really know what they're doing and they don't have enough knowledge, that kind of thing. I know that at my last job before I retired, running the Health Services Center at a university, I had six doctors, three nurse practitioners and the usual lab staff, etc., and I really got to intimately know what these people were thinking and doing and I could observe how they were treating people. And they were never referring out to chiropractors.

All the doctors I saw for my back were positive about my coming back to see you, enthusiastic, and thought it was a wise decision. They did warn me that it might help [but] it might not, of course. But they hadn't provided the answer either. The surgeon was not as enthusiastic, but had no objections at all and just said, "If this can help you, good."

But it had no effect on my decision to come here and work with you. You were the one who kept me coming back. Even though it's a long drive for me, it's been worth it. And I've never for a moment considered giving up. In fact, now I can't conceive of not having any chiropractic.

DR. PATON: *It's true that you can never really make a true correction given the effects of gravity on a scoliotic spine that's fused due to age-related arthritis. So we keep things as best aligned as we can. In the case of kids with scoliosis, sometimes they respond so incredibly that the scoliosis actually disappears. Medical doctors don't believe it, but it's true. And it's amazing what wellness adjustments—or maintenance adjustments—can do for your body once you get things stabilized.*

BRIAN: I was very comfortable coming once a week but you were right, that twice a week would be even better. The improvement has continued. And if you can keep me at this level, I'll be very pleased. My daughter, too, can't imagine ever stopping.

DR. PATON: *Thank you so much, Brian. Is there anything else you'd like to add?*

BRIAN: Well, only that I don't really know what chiropractors can do to get more respect for the profession—I've watched it in three different countries—but I think it's an effect of the doctors saying to their patients that they shouldn't try it. Just because doctors have a piece of paper on the wall doesn't mean they are really qualified, and I'm sure there are chiropractors like that, too. But I am not impressed at all with prescriptions and fancy lunches. I don't know whether chiropractors would ever want to write prescriptions…

DR. PATON: *Definitely not. When I feel someone needs a prescription, I refer them out to the orthopedic surgeon or to their primary care doctor. Say, for example, I find a patient has high blood pressure. My goal is to only temporarily get their blood pressure under control with medication so we can start them on adjustments, with an exercise and nutrition plan to get in shape until they can then get off the medication.*

Unfortunately, in America, most people are handed a prescription and no one really recommends for you to change your lifestyle.

BRIAN: Yes, people really don't take good care of themselves. And all those stories of politicians saying that the whole world is dying to get to America for medical care—Canadian care is certainly just as good. Even South African care was just as good. But now because of my experience with you, my opinion of chiropractic has changed totally.

The differences of chiropractic
Now that you know what chiropractic does, it's time to compare it to some other treatments. I regularly encounter questions about chiropractic and osteopathic care: whether there is any difference and, if there is any, exactly what it is.

Osteopathy, like chiropractic, is an approach to healthcare that emphasizes the role of the musculoskeletal system in the prevention and treatment of disease. In practice, this most commonly relates to musculoskeletal problems such as back and neck pain.

Andrew Taylor Still, M.D./D.O., is considered the father of osteopathic medicine and was the founder of the first college of osteopathic medicine in 1892. Apprentice to his father, also a physician, and a surgeon in the Union Army during the Civil War, Andrew Still ultimately became disillusioned with his medical counterparts, criticizing their misuse of common drugs.

Following the death of three of his children from spinal meningitis in 1864, Still concluded further that the orthodox medical practices of his day were frequently ineffective and sometimes harmful, and devoted the next ten years of his life to studying the human body and finding better ways to treat disease.

Based on philosophies that focus on the unity of all body parts and the musculoskeletal system as a key element of health, Still believed that medicine should offer the patient more, including osteopathic manipulative treatment. He believed in the body's inherent ability to heal itself and stressed preventive medicine, eating properly, and keeping fit.

On its Website, www.osteopathiecollege.com, the Canadian College of Osteopathy asserts that this methodology was proven to be successful with musculoskeletal issues and major diseases of Still's time, including TB, pneumonia, dysentery and typhoid fever.

So, osteopathy has a similar background to the development as chiropractic, doesn't it? They are both based on a physician's unwillingness to adhere to treatment guidelines provided by established medicine, and on a physician's belief in the body's inherent desire to heal itself.

Through the years, however, though chiropractic and osteopathic philosophies have remained similar, their methods and objectives have diverged significantly. Osteopathy, for example, uses many of the diagnostic procedures used in conventional medical assessment and diagnosis, and a wide variety of approaches to treatment. In essence, the objective of the osteopathic profession is the therapeutic assessment and treatment of diseases and ailments of various kinds, essentially identical to that of medicine.

Chiropractic, on the other hand, specifically "straight, non-therapeutic chiropractic" (versus "mixed" chiropractic, using a mixture of a chiropractor with a non-chiropractic matter, the older approach based on a split from the founding principles of chiropractic about a century ago), specializes in the manipulation of the spine exclusively, its roots firmly planted in the belief that when the body is in true balance, it will heal itself.

Today there are four main groups of chiropractors: traditional straights, objective straights, mixers, and reforms. All groups, except reforms, treat patients using a system based on the technique of subluxation.

Straight chiropractic deals with the particular, common situation called a vertebral subluxation. Essentially, adjusting (or correcting a vertebral subluxation) allows the spinal bone to return to its proper position by removing the breakdown of vital information transmitted through the nerves.

Although there is a procedure in osteopathy called "manipulation," in which various bones are moved—and this is likely why most people often compare chiropractic and osteopathy—the difference in the core objective between non-therapeutic straight chiropractic and osteopathy makes any meaningful comparison virtually impossible.

Specifically, and most critically, osteopathic manipulations are not directed toward the correction of vertebral subluxation, and so will not be applied with the same technical considerations or evaluated based upon the same analyses.

In terms of the actual manipulation itself, when it is performed by an osteopath it is more of a general overall mobilization/manipulation procedure at the site of injury/complaint and adjacent areas. The osteopath searches for fixations based on where pain is located and then regards the site of injury as a place where there is a lack of circulation, which dictates manipulation to enhance that circulation. Osteopathic manipulation cavitates, or "pops," vertebrae (spinal bones) in an effort to release those fixations. When these "non-specific" adjustments are made, often the patient's pain will recede, but only temporarily.

One of the reasons this occurs is because when the bones are "popped," endorphins are released, creating a sense of feeling good naturally. Unfortunately, it's a quick but not a permanent fix, because the true innate or *qi* (life flow or balance) has not been restored—and that's what it really takes to improve a patient's condition over the long term. Chiropractic manipulation, on the other hand, is an extremely specific and precise adjustment.

Another significant difference between osteopathy and chiropractic—and one not to be minimized—is the fact that osteopaths have the license to prescribe medication. I personally have noted over the years an unfortunate trend relative to the practice of prescribing more drugs as a first line of treatment, by osteopaths also. Many, however, refer to chiropractors because their medical education relates the condition of the spine and overall healthcare as a direct relationship.

Although many osteopaths hold an open mind with regard to chiropractic treatment, there are also many who have seemingly lost touch with the original osteopathic philosophy that the condition of the spine and its balance is a direct reflection of a person's health.

Eastern medicine: Acupuncture

Like chiropractic, Eastern medicine appreciates this holistic approach.

In acupuncture, the focus is on the body's *meridians*, called *jing luo* in Chinese, meaning "channels" or "conduits," which are like the meridians that circle the Earth. These invisible channels circulate *qi* (pronounced *chee*) throughout the body. There are many places where the *qi* of the channels rise close to the surface of the body, and these are the acupuncture "points." There are twelve main meridians, and numerous minor ones, that form the energetic network of channels throughout the body.

In acupuncture, each meridian is related to, and named after, an organ or function. The main ones are the lung, kidney, gall bladder, stomach, spleen, heart, small intestine, large intestine, liver, urinary bladder, *san jiao* ("triple warmer") and pericardium (heart protector or circulation/sex meridian).

Simply put, picture two rooms connected by a door. One room is empty and the other is filled with water. Balancing meridians with acupuncture is like opening the door between the two rooms. Water from the full room will flow into the empty one and the larger structure (consisting of both rooms) will balance itself out perfectly. The human body, the Earth, the universe—everything around us requires balance. Without it, we have disease.

Without the inherent balance of the Earth's gravitational pull, we would be floating in the atmosphere. The sun is large enough to have gravitational pull on the Earth, which keeps it in perfect rotation. Even though we can't feel gravity, it's part of the natural flow of the universe. It's the same way with our natural state of innate or *qi*. We don't think about it ordinarily but when something feels wrong, we know it. It's when we feel *out* of balance that we feel the need to *re*balance.

Our physical bodies need to stay rooted, balanced, in a deep, inherent way, and that means more than taking a pill to bring it back down to Earth. Taking drugs is like leaving the door closed and then complaining you have no water. For that matter, why take drugs when most of the time the answer is as easy as opening the door (and your mind)?

I have to admit to being pretty typical in terms of following a conventional path for most of my life until I started learning about chiropractic. When I entered the field of sports medicine, I never considered alternative styles of healing as part of my palette. As chiropractic care proved to be more and more useful as a tool to help my patients, however, I began to be more open-minded about techniques I'd heard about but never considered. Acupuncture is one of those tools.

I also have to admit that I, too, had bought into the powerful system that was giving all "alternative treatments" a bad name—and not by people who have experienced them. It took me a while to discern why there was such a profound resistance towards potentially helpful treatment alternatives, but the reality of the situation makes perfect sense. Medical lobbyists are in the back pockets of the AMA, which lobbies for the drug companies. Why wouldn't the AMA try to squash alternative care in an attempt to monopolize healthcare and keep our focus on specialized, non-holistic, disease-oriented approaches, with drug therapies as the only viable answer?

I recently attended a class presented by Dr. Richard Yennie (Doctor of Chiropractic, Diplomate in Acupuncture [NCCA], President of the Acupuncture Society of America), who revealed just how far the system has been willing to go to ensure its safety from the threat of "outside" methodologies.

One example is of an initiative put on the table for the sole purpose of putting all acupuncturists out of business by insisting that acupuncture is a surgical procedure in order to bring it under the auspices of general Westernized healthcare. This is a perfect example of how the establishment wants to have it both ways. How can acupuncture be a "surgical procedure" on the one hand and at the same time be "pseudo-science" and "quackery"?

As a chiropractor, I treat researchers who work for those same drug companies; I treat oncologists, primary care physicians, nurses, pharmacists—all of whom realize the benefits of chiropractic because they've chosen to be open-minded. As society begins to accept—and embrace—alternative methodologies due to their patients' insistence, even some hospitals and treatment facilities are jumping on board. They realize that denying the benefits of these therapies not only puts them at risk of losing their patients' loyalties, but also puts them at risk where it hurts the most—their bottom line.

Sadly, though, the individuals working in medical professions where alternative therapies are consistently overlooked are the ones who suffer the most. Only when they risk going outside the system by coming to see someone like me do they get to experience other potential, rewarding solutions.

My own experience with acupuncture

For me personally, opening up to the possibility of new ways of thinking and treating my patients has been revolutionary. Taking classes has been inspirational and instrumental in the direction of my practice and, I believe, its success. Acupuncture is one area I hesitated (or, more accurately, loathed) to enter, however, mostly because of my hatred for needles.

It's true. I hate needles.

It's hard to admit out loud, but when I see them, I actually feel faint. When I have blood drawn I have to lie down. Not an auspicious beginning for someone interested in how using needles can correct the flow of the body's innate intelligence! But because I could no longer ignore the relief so many of my patients were achieving from acupuncture, I knew I needed to see what it was all about for myself.

Dr. Yennie started by showing us the needles used in acupuncture treatments. It was hard for me to even look at them, but when I did, the first thing I saw was how tiny they were, much smaller than I'd imagined them in my mind. Then one of the instructors asked each of us to put one in a certain point in his/her own arm. I was terrified and thought I'd pass out but I forced myself to do it. Each needle is so tiny that it's stored in a pipette to prevent it from bending when it hits your skin. When it didn't hurt, I was shocked.

So I tapped it in and pulled the pipette off. No pain! I stood there looking at the needle in my skin and didn't know how to react. I knew it felt painless, but my stomach was still telling me I felt queasy just looking at it.

The instructor said, "I want you to feel the *qi*, manipulate the needle; this is what makes a good acupuncturist. Push it in further until you feel a tingling or pressure, and that's the *qi*, the flow of energy." I wanted to feel that flow so badly...

Then I got light-headed. I quietly raised my hand and one of the instructors came over. I said, "I don't want to embarrass myself but I'm going to faint if I push this needle in any farther. But I really want to feel the *qi*." She reached over and I reacted by jumping and pushing her hand away. All she was going to do was pull the needle out—which she proceeded to do. Then I felt disappointed because I had wanted to experience the *qi*.

I sat quietly, experiencing a whole range of emotions about what had just happened.

I had been experiencing back pain due to sleeping in an awkward position on the flight for this class in Kansas City. The low back pain was disrupting my *qi*, the innate intelligence was manifesting in my back pain.

Since I started regular adjustments, I experience little if any back pain anymore, but at that time the regular discomfort was interrupting my day-to-day life. The class had just started the day before, and I had already received several adjustments and electrical acupressure (called auriculotherapy), which helped temporarily, but I still had back pain. I was frustrated and uncomfortable, believing that my problem was a disruption in *qi* due to an out-of-place lower lumbar spine.

I will never forget what happened next.

After lunch, the teacher introduced a doctor by the name of Dr. Gao, a Chinese acupuncturist. Apparently Dr. Quizhi Gao has practiced traditional Chinese medicine for over twenty-five years and has thirty years' experience as a Qigong Practitioner and Instructor. In 1992, Dr. Gao moved to Kansas, where he established his practice with an emphasis in acupuncture, Qigong, *Tuina Anmo* (Asian bodywork) and herbal medicine, then founded the Kansas College of Chinese Medicine in Witchita in the fall of 1996.

I sat back to listen, still unhappy with what had happened that morning and uncomfortable in the chair due to my back pain, when—lo and behold—out of the clear blue, Dr. Gao said, "Who has neck pain and who has low back pain?"

I immediately raised my hand, hoping—and assuming—that I would be volunteering for some sort of acupressure treatment. In other words: no needles. Two of us raised our hands and were called up to the front of the room. In the meantime, I saw Dr. Gao taking out his needles. "Oh, no," I thought, not really wanting to be up there. I didn't have the nerve to return to my seat, however, and began to get lightheaded, feeling worse and worse as I watched in dismay while Dr. Gao worked on the other volunteer, who had neck pain.

Then came my turn.

I quietly asked Dr. Gao—desperately trying not to embarrass myself—"Can I please kneel down? I might pass out. I don't like needles."

"You don't like needles?" he asked, and the whole class chuckled as one. The doctor then said, "It will be okay, it won't hurt. Why don't you sit down on this chair?"

I put my arm on the table, but was really jumpy—moving my feet, covering my eyes, gritting my teeth. I was just plain nervous, waiting for the pain. Dr. Gao could see my discomfort. "I tell you what," he said. "We'll just do specific points and I'll work with my finger."

He began to work with his thumb only. He flexed my back and applied pressure at each of three points, asking which hurt worst: 1, 2 or 3. They all felt the same. They hurt at about 20 degrees of flexion, and caused pain to the right. He worked a few points and then I could bend forward to a greater extent. At that point, I just said, "Okay, give me the needle. I'm not going to step off this stage until then…I'm going to be a man about this."

"We don't want you to faint," said Dr. Gao.

"No, stick it in there right now. Whatever you need to do." I heard the class laughing in the background but nothing would stop me now.

"We could continue this way…it's working," he said.

"Doctor, stick that needle in there right now because I'm not going to deal the rest of the year with my friends in the audience making fun of me about this." I grit my teeth.

"It's not going to hurt," he said, then poked the needle in and pulled off the pipette. "Done!" Then he actually manipulated the needle and tapped it with his finger; at that moment, I felt the most amazing thing. I felt the *qi*! They had described it earlier as a feeling of warmth and pressure in the spot around the needle, and that's exactly what it was.

"How do you feel?" Dr. Gao asked.

I bent forward without any pain.

"How do you feel?" he repeated.

"I can't believe it," I admitted. "I'm not feeling pain in my back. But what's really cool is that I feel this pressure in my hand and the pressure is slowly moving up my arm. It's very warm…"

"That's the *qi*."

I saw a lot of envy on the faces of the people in the audience because they hadn't felt it—and I knew I had experienced something amazing: how a truly gifted acupuncturist will manipulate the needle to achieve *qi*.

I immediately set myself a personal goal: When I included acupuncture in my practice, I would do much more than take a test for certification. I would dedicate myself to learning how to manipulate the needle to help my patients achieve true *qi*.

Schools of thought

There are three schools of thought regarding acupuncture. The first school is classic, called the "yin and the yang." The second one is made up of "skeptics," who maintain that acupuncture (a practice already thousands of years old) is a "pseudoscience." The third consists of "integrationists," a growing group in the United States that appreciates Western medicine, acupuncture, chiropractic, and other less conventional treatments.

The idea of harmony and balance is the basis for yin and yang, the principle that each person is governed by opposing, but complementary, forces. This principle is central to all Chinese thought and is believed to affect everything in the universe, including ourselves. Yin and yang are the opposites that make the whole and cannot exist without each other. Because nothing is ever completely one or the other, they must exist as opposites, such as hot and cold, light and dark, or above and below.

This is true for all aspects of our lives. *In utero*, for example, we exist in a naturally balanced state. The birth process is what starts the disruption of this state and it happens so fast in the United States—using cesarean sections, clamps, forceps, anything to rush the process along—that we don't let nature take its course. If you've ever seen the actual birth process, you know that in order to bring the baby's shoulders out either through a C-section or through the birth canal, the head is used as a lever. If you recall, that's exactly what happened to my son, and it is one of the reasons I came to write this book.

What I now know is that my son's *qi* was completely disrupted during the birth process. I don't really blame the doctor; that's the way he was taught. Frankly, I don't know if there's any traditional medical practice in the United States that allows—helps—a baby to be born with the least amount of disruption to the *qi* possible.

In my son's case, it wasn't that he needed acupuncture specifically, but that the disruption of innate occurred when his spine was misaligned during the birth process. Yin suddenly didn't equal yang, hence his "illness." Again, the medical establishment immediately headed down the entirely wrong path by attempting to use drugs, which would have only masked his symptoms, asking not *why* he might be experiencing what they felt was "acid reflux" but only how to treat its symptoms. I thank God every day that I knew enough as a chiropractor to react the way I did in adjusting my son's spine.

Because Western medicine only studies the physical body, it is missing a vast amount of knowledge that focuses on how the energy flows and how the mind can change the body. Even the anatomical charts of the human body in Eastern medicine differ radically from those of Western medicine, particularly in the United States. Eastern medical charts reveal the pathways of the meridians first and foremost.

When was *qi* or innate created? When the universe was created…and it continues to this day. I personally believe it's a slap in the face to the powers that created this universe for Western medicine to deny this body of knowledge.

The body's life force
Our bodies function via electrical impulses. Without them, we cannot live—we pass on and leave this green Earth for a more heavenly place.

Electricity is normally produced by power plants or generators, yet, amazingly, our bodies can generate it for free all on its own. The body accomplishes this by lining up ions such as potassium and sodium in just the right way to elicit an electrical impulse.

Most of the time we can't see or feel this electricity, although it can be measured with EKGs, but there is some electricity created by the human body that we *can* see. Static electricity occurs when our bodies develop an increased electrical charge and then we touch something metallic. Then, sometimes, we can see a small spark when our bodies charge up to 400-500 volts. If the static electricity is enough to make our hair stand up, it is at least 1,000 V or volts, and it would not be uncommon to hear, see *and* feel that charge.

Some electrical impulses are strong; others are weak. The electrical impulse that causes the heart to pump is around 90-100 mV or millivolts. The brain utilizes electricity generated by the body to send commands to every single organ, gland and muscle so that we function properly. The amount of electricity required to make a nerve carry an impulse in the body is also around 100 mV.

The art of acupuncture is concerned with these natural bioelectrical magnetic pathways of the human body—not enough current to start your car engine, but certainly enough to keep our bodies functioning properly.

What is true health?

Health is not the absence of illness the way so many think, but rather the expression of our own individual innate.

In Eastern medicine, because there is such an appreciation for massage therapy as a science, the student must study for five full years prior to certification. Massage is not just to help you feel good at the moment; it's an attempt to restore the *qi*. If the problem with the *qi* is that there's a misalignment of the spine, that's a job for another practitioner (a chiropractor). After that treatment, massage therapy can work on restoring and promoting the flow. In China, the emphasis is getting it all to work together.

The stages of disease

The human body responds to disruptions in the *qi* in four stages, which ultimately results in disease or illness.

Stage One: The original cause, a disruption in the *qi* or in the innate, which occurs due to an injury or some other stressor.

Stage Two: Functional disorder takes place—lack of motion, for example. There's no pain yet, but things aren't working the way they should. It could be a dysfunctional spine that starts the degenerative process.

Stage Three: Symptoms, which are what finally get people to the doctor. Most go directly to the medical doctor, who helps disguise the original problem by covering up the symptoms. Neither the functional disorder nor the original cause is addressed; there is suppression of the faulty circuit, the innate imbalance.

Stage Four: Organ failure. If the original imbalance is not effectively sought out and treated, the disease will progress until it will be difficult, if not impossible, to treat successfully.

When people come into my chiropractic office and are asked how long they've been suffering, more likely than not they'll answer two to three weeks. On average, it takes two to three weeks of pain before they are driven to do something about it, which often includes making an appointment. Prior to this, most of them have been covering up their pain with drugs for a much longer period of time. They come in when the drugs stop working or when their bodies have become immune to them.

People don't usually last too long with pain and suffering, but that's one of the last stages of disease. Bone spurs, spinal degeneration, disk degeneration, etc. take years to be created, not weeks. By the time the symptoms present, these conditions have been manifesting silently for five to ten years!

One of the keys is to stop looking at healthcare as the absence of illness or pain. Just because it doesn't hurt—yet—doesn't mean you shouldn't go to an acupuncturist, chiropractor, or massage

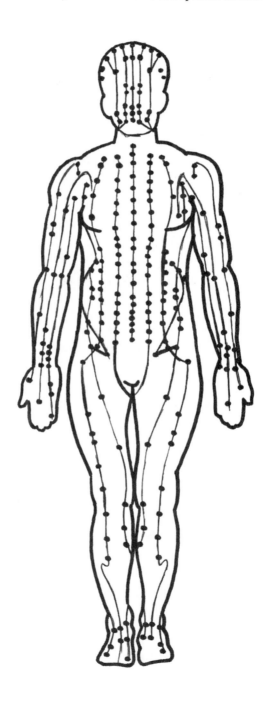

therapist. Going regularly *keeps* you healthy! We need to look at healthcare as promoting the proper flow of innate intelligence, the proper flow of *qi*, to keep us in balance and healthy.

Did you know that in ancient China people would STOP paying the doctor when they got sick? That's the kind of real healthcare we need!

When *qi* flows freely through the meridians, a balanced, healthy body results; if the energy becomes blocked, stagnated or weakened, physical, mental or emotional ill health can result. Imbalances are caused by any number of emotional responses (such as excess anger, over-excitement, self-pity, deep grief and fear), environmental factors (such as cold, damp/humidity, wind, dryness, and heat) or excesses (such as wrong diet, too much sex, overwork and too much exercise).

To restore the balance or *qi*, the acupuncturist stimulates the acupuncture points that will counteract that imbalance. For example, if your *qi* is stagnant, the practitioner will choose the specific points to stimulate it. If the *qi* is too cold, specific points will be chosen to warm it; if too weak, points will be chosen to strengthen it, etc. In this way, acupuncture can effectively rebalance the energy system and restore health or prevent the development of disease. Because the points run along the body's meridians, the ones chosen may not necessarily be (and are often not) at the site(s) of the patient's symptoms.

Techniques of acupuncture and chiropractic
There is an interesting correlation between acupuncture techniques and chiropractic techniques. As I mentioned, a good acupuncturist will manipulate the needle by turning it to find the place to achieve true *qi*. A chiropractor uses specific adjustments in the same way.

It is my understanding that acupuncturists use needles 3-7 out of 10 times; the rest of the time, they use electrical acupuncture or acupressure (applying microcurrents of electricity to those same points on the meridians for stimulation).

One of the most important attributes of these kinds of therapies is how they work together. For example, when I left Kansas City after my volunteer acupuncture treatment, my pain did return to a small degree. But the acupuncture had relaxed my back to the point where I was now able to be adjusted, and accept that adjustment on a physical level more successfully. My spine had been locked up and was now unlocked. It was moving like butter and by the time I had my adjustment when I got back home, I could feel the release from the gentle, light pressure adjustment I received.

So, does every person who sees an acupuncturist need to see a chiropractor or vice versa? No. But getting checked monthly by one or the other can help you stay really healthy, and the opposite is also true. Once a subluxation or blockage has begun, eventually there will be some type of manifestation—spasms, headaches, acid reflux, disease, some symptoms to reveal that blockage or imbalance. Maintaining an open flow of *qi* through adjustment or acupuncture can help us achieve—*and maintain*—true health.

Acupuncture is an important adjunct to chiropractic care, which is one of the critical five factors of health: chiropractic adjustments (along with possible acupuncture and massage therapy), a positive mental attitude, exercise, proper nutrition and proper sleep.

These five factors implemented over the long term keep the *qi* flowing and keep us consistently healthy.

CHAPTER NINE

CHILDREN AND CHIROPRACTIC CARE

Chiropractic and a lifelong commitment to health

Chiropractic is so much more than treatment for neck and back pain! That's what my patients realize after bringing their sons and daughters, as well as mothers, fathers and friends, in for treatment of all kinds of problems. But, in truth, a majority of the cases I see are indeed caused by spinal subluxation, a misalignment of the vertebra that causes pressure on a nerve.

As I said, the first subluxation we ever experience occurs as early as birth. Since there are so many opportunities for misalignments to occur during the modern birth process (with C-sections, forceps and all that accompanies it), it is extremely unlikely to come across a baby born today who would not need some kind of adjustment to compensate for the results on the spine.

And that's just the beginning. Children are moving from the moment of birth; from there, it's on to crawling, walking and falling on a regular basis. So how do we know when and what to realign?

The signs of misalignment

For children, many signs of misalignment manifest as illness. Are they getting earaches, ear infections, sore throats? Are they hyper-active, colicky? Do they scream relentlessly for no apparent reason? Do they spit up more food or milk than they keep down? Do they get colds often? Is their posture awkward? Is one foot splayed out farther than the other? Is one pant leg shorter than the other? As they get older, are they complaining of headaches or allergies?

Many teenagers experiencing headaches and bipolar disorder are currently being treated with Topamax, a drug for seizures and migraines. But, in fact, many of these so-called "inexplicable" symptoms are merely representations of a spinal misalignment that need attention. Bring them to a chiropractor *before* putting them on drugs!

Scoliosis and chiropractic

Scoliosis is another fairly common condition I see, where the spine curves from side to side (left to right, *not* front to back) as opposed to the more natural position of a straight line. Sometimes the bones in a scoliotic spine rotate slightly, making the waist or shoulders appear uneven, but contrary to common belief, scoliosis does not come from slouching, sitting in awkward positions, or sleeping on an old mattress.

Some forms of scoliosis are classified as congenital (caused by vertebral anomalies present at birth); others are referred to as idiopathic (of unknown cause). Although the cause may be listed as idiopathic, chiropractors know that this is not the case. The cause is usually a misaligned spinal vertebra—and the result of a vertebra that misaligns or rotates out of place is a compensating curvature. Idiopathic scoliosis is therefore usually best treated by a chiropractor. It's usually a simple fix: correct the misaligned vertebra and the scoliosis will straighten.

I have treated too many children to count whose parents were beside themselves when they saw the pre-treatment x-ray with scoliosis and a post-treatment x-ray with a straight spine. Unfortunately too many medical doctors will dispute this and claim that scoliosis is not correctable, so they "keep an eye on it" as the child grows. I want to scream every time I hear that statement about keeping an eye on it; in the meantime, it's not getting any better by itself! All I can think is, "That poor child."

Occasionally, scoliotic curvatures in the spine are caused by uneven growth of a child's legs. As a child grows, one leg may grow slightly faster than the other, which, in turn, causes one hip to be higher than the other. The body's response is to try to compensate— it does not want to stand crookedly, so it will naturally form a curvature in the spine to compensate for the shorter leg.

Basically, the body is attempting to achieve the "righting" reflex (also called *static reflex*), which is any reflex that tends to bring the body into normal position spatially and resist forces acting to displace from this normal position. Simply put, our brains will do whatever it has to do to our bodies to attempt to make our eyes parallel with the horizon.

On occasion, as the child continues to grow, the bone growth of the shorter leg will eventually catch up. But even though the hips level out, the spinal curvature persists. Fortunately, this type of curvature is correctable with a safe chiropractic adjustment, and because the ligaments are still pliable, children are often correctable to nearly 100%.

When the spine is curved to the point of scoliosis, symptoms can include uneven musculature on one side of the spine, a rib "hump" and/or a prominent shoulder blade (more pronounced when the child bends over), uneven hip and shoulder levels, asymmetric size or location of a breast (in females), an unequal distance between the arms and body, clothes that do not 'hang right,' or, the most common symptoms, seemingly "uneven" leg lengths due to any of the previous.

In this situation of a "functional" short leg due to a pelvic misalignment, we can add a lift to the short leg (to the shoe) temporarily and hope it catches up in a growth spurt and balances out, along with adjusting the spine to promote a straighter, more balanced line. In the extremely rare case that the legs never reach a balanced state, some children will unfortunately have uncorrectable scoliosis, but please see a chiropractor to find out if this is the case.

In conclusion, although scoliosis in children is almost 100% correctable, adult scoliosis is *not*. That's why it's so important to correct this condition before the child becomes an adult. It's so crucial to take them early to a reputable chiropractor, someone you know has seen children with success. I think you might be surprised that, if you ask neighbors and friends, you'll find there are quite a number who go to chiropractors for treatment.

If your child has been diagnosed with scoliosis and your pediatrician tells you not to bring him to a chiropractor, I strongly suggest you find another pediatrician. I know how difficult this can be to hear and I only ask my readers to consider their options. Doing nothing and "keeping an eye on things"—i.e., *not* considering utilizing chiropractic care for this type of condition—can do a lot more damage than proceeding with an open mind and correcting the problem.

As I have indicated throughout this book, I make many referrals to medical doctors when a patient's need is beyond the scope of chiropractic care. I believe strongly that it's up to me to recognize when the patient requires the care of someone other than myself or needs a type of treatment I am unable to provide, and I expect other medical professionals to do the same. After all, we should all be working together in the best interest of your child.

Bedwetting

I also want to make a short comment here about enuresis, better known as bedwetting. It is a common condition that upsets many parents as well as children, but it is a condition that can be treated easily and effectively in most cases.

It is a little known fact that chiropractors treat bedwetting in children, but my office has a nearly perfect success rate in this area.

Many times, it is when the middle lumbar vertebra, L3, is out of alignment that bladder control weakens. In these cases, L3 is impinging on the nerve that supplies the bladder and the muscles around the urethra, which control the closing of the urethra—and an adjustment can work wonders. Using medication for bladder control, on the other hand, is often simply an attempt to affect a symptom whose root cause is something else altogether.

The results I've had with treating enuresis have been phenomenal. Out of all the successful cases I've had with this disorder, I have treated only one child who did not respond, for unknown reasons, and was very saddened and frustrated at not having had success with this young boy since I've seen so many other parents thrilled with their children's response to chiropractic care.

Chiropractic care and infants

By now, you know all about how I adjusted my three-day-old son Nicholas in the hospital. You've read about how the birth process is inherently disruptive to a newborn's physiological well-being. Yet you still know how unusual it would be for a hospital to consider infant spinal manipulations as part of their program of treatment.

I sincerely hope that in writing about this, I will encourage my readers to spread the word about the almost miraculous benefits infant adjustments can have—on a variety and wide spectrum of symptoms. If this book helps one child by keeping him from lengthy drug therapies, antibiotic courses or painful treatments, I will be an even happier person indeed.

How do you know when a baby needs an adjustment?

I know that for some readers, it will be difficult to accept my adjusting an infant. But that's just when a newborn needs it after the traumatic entry into the world through the typical birth process. Health problems can start that early—moments into life—but can also be averted or corrected in a timely fashion.

The birth process is not an easy one, whether it's a vaginal birth or a C-section, because birthing requires a baby to be pulled, pushed and prodded to exit the womb and enter a wholly different environment. Sometimes the doctor will have to pull the baby's head out first then use the head as a lever to pry the shoulders out. Sometimes forceps are required to pull the head out with enough force to get the shoulders out, too. I have a friend who told me that when his baby was born, the doctor put so much force behind the forceps in order to pull the baby out that she actually slipped right off her chair. So it doesn't take much to imagine that a baby might have difficulties brought on by such forceful handling.

On the other hand, adjusting a baby is an infinitely gentler procedure. The pressure involved is so light as to be almost unnoticeable. To give you an idea of the level of pressure, take your finger and place the tip of it on a table in front of you. Push down on your finger *just enough to blanch the tip of your fingernail* (so that it starts to turn white). The pressure you exert and feel just *before* the tip of your fingernail turns white is approximately the amount of pressure used to adjust an infant.

Compare this to the amount of pressure caused by the birth process itself, along with the all the pushing, pulling and trauma. Frankly, it's no contest.

An example of infant chiropractic care

When Janice came to me for shoulder adjustments, I was unaware that her granddaughter was having problems with colic. One of the issues, unfortunately, is that people just don't think about chiropractic in terms of their small children or infants, and are not prone to bring it up in the natural course of conversation. In this case, Janice had been coming to me long enough that our conversations covered a wider range of topics than usual—and I am grateful that they did.

She told me that her baby granddaughter was suffering from colic and seemed to be gasping for air. She'd been such a happy baby that her family was upset by her recent obvious distress and didn't know what to do. I told her to bring her in and I'd see what I could do to help. The following interview covers the issue of the baby's chiropractic care:

DR. PATON: *What was your family's reaction when you told them you wanted to bring in your granddaughter for chiropractic treatment here?*

JANICE: They weren't happy. My daughter and husband said, "He'll know more than the pediatrician does?" I had to explain to them that it's a totally different way of treating the symptoms. They were uncomfortable about it, but I insisted I could trust you and that you might be able to help.

DR. PATON: *At this point, the baby's been adjusted three times. Have you noticed changes in her condition?*

JANICE: Definitely. She seems like her old self again; she's happy-go-lucky, the way she used to be. We're not having any problems at all. What I would like to ask you is why she is not having the gas anymore.

DR. PATON: *The best way I can explain it is by explaining just how important the connection is between the brain and the spinal cord. Your brain and spinal cord control and coordinate every single process in your entire body. So if you break your neck by diving into the shallow end of a pool or falling from a horse, everything stops—everything:*

kidney function, leg movement, sometimes breathing capability. Breaking one's neck means a severe impingement in the spine, sometimes so severe that it partially severs the spinal cord.

Of course, this is the extreme case to illustrate what can happen, but the point is that spinal impingement can cause all sorts of conditions. In less severe cases, there will still be functionality, but the pressure on the nerve or nerves will still cause some type of negative reaction.

In a baby with colic, what is almost always the case is that the nerve has been impinged at the level of T6, and that is the nerve that relates to the stomach. Stomachs react to this kind of impingement just the way necks and backs do, along with glands and organs—they don't get painful necessarily, but they become dysfunctional. Neck and back impingement can lead to numbness down the arms or headaches, but instead the stomach reacts in its own way, and when the stomach becomes dysfunctional there is no sign of symptom other than the colic.

Because the stomach is a muscle, when it goes into spasm, all the extra gas (gastric air bubbles) gets pinched and everything slows down. The same thing can happen with the intestines. Everyone has gas bubbles, but when you follow them on x-rays you can see where there is a backup. It's almost like a shoestring has been tied around the intestine because you can see all the gas backing up and it's actually swelling. I can see that the person will have constipation or gas pains. At that point I can guess that T12 and L1 are both places that will need adjustment because those are the nerves that go to the intestines.

So, in a baby it's either going to be T6 or T12 and L1. I check those in every single infant I see—and it works.

JANICE: When she drank, it always seemed like it could not go down fast enough. Was that from air bubbles? She could only drink so much before it was backing up…like it couldn't go anywhere. The baby was starving but she shouldn't keep anything down; she'd keep spitting it up.

DR. PATON: *No, that's a different situation. That's actually the sphincter, which is also connected to the T5-T6 nerves. Sphincters are muscles and intestines are muscles, so they spasm just as your neck and lower back do. When they spasm, they close up and things can't* *happen as quickly. When you take the pressure off those nerves, the muscles calm down and can function normally.*

In medicine, they would say you have IBS—Irritable Bowel Syndrome—and offer a medication to relax your intestinal muscles. It is my feeling that this does not at all address the real cause of the problem.

JANICE: I know that parents don't know what else to do. They think the baby isn't hungry or is allergic to milk or something…you know *something* is wrong. But I don't think they've ever heard of getting a baby adjusted. I was to the point where I was going to bring her in on my own. I finally said to them, "That is a child in pain. She needs help."

DR. PATON: *Do you think the people you know are more receptive to chiropractic now?*

JANICE: Definitely. They were not before. Nobody was. I told them I was having my five-month-old baby adjusted at the chiropractor's office and they looked at me, like, *okay*…but now they're all saying, "She's the old Olivia again."

As this conversation shows, chiropractic is definitely one of the lifelong factors that should be considered to maintain consistent good health—from granddaughter to grandmother, from infancy to adulthood.

There are, however, four other factors that we need to explore in order to keep the body in balance—which is not only the ultimate goal of chiropractic care, but also the key to physical health and the ideal state of everything in the universe.

CHAPTER TEN

EXERCISE: THE SECOND FACTOR OF HEALTH

The five factors of health

Our children don't eat junk food. There are no sugary cereals in our closet.

They get adjusted regularly, eat right, drink healthy drinks, and they've never had an ear infection or a sore throat. We're doing something right here, and my goal is to share the information with everyone I possibly can.

With that said, if you still believe that junk food, lack of exercise and drugs are the way to go after reading this book, then I will support *your right* to have those beliefs and make your own decisions. However, I will never be able to support those *decisions* themselves regarding how to live a healthy life.

By now, you know how I feel about a lot of the problems that face our society today: rising healthcare costs, our focus on illness over wellness, pressure by the drug companies to use more and more drugs, the medical establishment's determined efforts to snuff out alternative treatment options, just to name a few. But I hope I've also made it clear that there are many, *many* things we can do to change the way we live in order to make our lives happier and healthier.

In my years as a chiropractic practitioner, I have seen many patients come to me in pain, struggling to understand how they got to that point where nothing seems to help and no one seems to be offering a solution. It is for these people that I wrote this book. But I also wrote it for those of you simply looking for a new way of doing things, a new way of approaching your life and your health in order to access the kind of balanced existence you always knew was possible, but never knew how to achieve.

Now that you know about chiropractic, the first factor of health, let's look at the other things you can improve to change your life, the other important factors.

We'll start with exercise. Consistent exercise is something that very few people actually want to do. I can relate.

It can be really, *really* tough to exercise when your life gets busy. It's often the first thing we think we can afford to miss when other responsibilities vie for our attention. But, in reality, exercise is one of those critical aspects of a fully functional life. It helps us feel good about ourselves, our appearance and the world around us.

The third factor of good health is good nutrition. We all know how difficult that one can be, given our pervasive environment of fast food and easy fixin's. MSG, additives, pesticides, hormones, antibiotics—all are part of the typical American diet. In fact, it's virtually impossible to buy food in a regular supermarket or restaurant that has not been laced with one or more detrimental substances. Later, we will talk about the effects some of these substances have on our food and on our health, and how to find foods that contribute to our well-being instead.

Sleep, the fourth of five factors of good health, has been denigrated by many to a low rung on the ladder of luxuries in life. But without consistent, *good* sleep, human beings are virtually incapable of living in a meaningful way. We will talk about how sleep habits have changed over the years, how the Internet affects these patterns, why we need sleep, how much, and how to get it.

Last, but certainly not least, is a positive attitude, the fifth element for an overall strong, healthy system. Do not underestimate the power of the mind to overcome adversity and live with good health in our daily lives.

When these factors come together, you will *feel* the effects. You will have achieved the balance necessary for a healthy, happy life for yourself and your family. What could be more important?

There's more to exercise than meets the eye

"Exercise" is a word that many people avoid, never mind putting it into practice. But along with the physical benefits of exercise are many more that contribute to emotional and overall well-being. For some, getting out in nature on a hiking trail is all they need to face another week at the office. For others, going to the gym every day not only provides social interaction but counterbalances work-days spent at desks, staring at computer screens. Whatever your situation, exercise is one of the most necessary tools toward building health and a balanced body.

So why is it so hard for so many people to start an exercise program—and follow through on it? First of all, let me reassure you that it's not necessarily because you're "lazy" or there's an exercise gene that you were inconveniently born without.

Of course, there are some people who thrive on athleticism from an early age, and for those people the thought of living without regular exercise is anathema. But the majority of people across the country have a difficult time even beginning an exercise program, regardless of body type or size. There are a number of reasons for this tendency to put off exercising—especially if we haven't taken care of ourselves all along.

"I can't exercise because it's hard on my joints."

I often recommend jogging to people who want to start exercising. Their reaction is often, "But isn't it hard on the joints?" The answer is this: If you're in alignment, the likelihood of abnormal wear and tear (and/or pain) is highly unlikely.

If you are *out* of alignment, however, abnormal wear and tear is likely, if not the norm. That's the reason many people get arthritis—what we call unilateral osteoarthritis, in which one joint (the knee, for example) of two is affected. The misalignment causes abnormal wear and tear (on one side, not the other), which causes degeneration of the joint, which then causes pain. (This is in contrast to rheumatoid arthritis, which takes place bilaterally and occurs less often.)

Unfortunately, by the time people come into my office with pain, x-rays often show years of arthritic buildup. The symptom (the pain) is always the last to arrive in the disease process. Once arthritis is there, the damage has been done.

So, before you embark on an exercise routine (the second factor of health), it is important to get chiropractic care (the first factor).

Exercise and the pathways of energy

It is common knowledge in the medical community that our body's biochemical pathways sustain life by generating the energy we need. Understanding aspects of these processes and how they work can help us live in a way that promotes the best health possible.

One of the critical ways our pathways sustain us is by breaking down energy sources such as glucose so that we can use it to thrive. But, contrary to what many people believe, the body doesn't automatically break down the substances we ingest or funnel them along the correct paths to achieve the most positive end results—we need to train it to do so. This can most easily be explained in terms of exercise.

The way most people miss the boat when they exercise is that they're trying to exercise their bodies, not their pathways. Furthermore, in sedentary people, the pathways remain virtually untrained; they tire easily because the energy they burn is being turned directly into lactic acid, which makes muscles hurt and ache.

Let's go through the important process of how energy is used by our bodies.

The glycolytic pathway / Krebs cycle

The pathway we're going to focus on is called the glycolytic pathway and the Krebs cycle, or the citric acid cycle. The Krebs cycle is basically a sequence of reactions in living organisms in which oxidation of acetic acid provides energy for storage.

Glycolysis is the process through which glucose (better known as sugar) enters our cells, gets broken down and enters our bloodstream. Most of our energy (for our brain and muscle tissue) primarily comes from burning glucose, a simple sugar (monosaccharide) derived from carbohydrates (or "carbs"). When carbs are metabolized, they become sugar.

When our bodies burn glucose for energy, ironically, we get free energy back. Let's say you have a special car that runs on three fuels:

glucose, fat, and protein. This car also has three different fuel tanks, each for the appropriate fuel. We need to pump the fuel to the right tank so it can be utilized.

The "fat" fuel corresponds to the tank farthest away from its engine and in the lowest position, so energy must be spent via a pump to get the fuel to the engine. This is the most difficult form to utilize for energy to power our car.

Our "protein" fuel is made of amino acids, the key building blocks of the body, and its tank is one step closer to being able to power our car. It is one level above the fat fuel tank, but the fuel still has to go through a process—a change in its chemical structure—to turn into usable energy, meaning energy must be spent to burn it.

Our last form of fuel is "glucose." The glucose fuel tank sits at a point higher and farther away than the other two tanks, higher even than the engine. This gives it the capacity of flowing downward; aided by the force of gravity, you don't even need a pump to access it. Our glucose fuel also has its own special feature: when this specific fuel is burned, the engine automatically connects to several batteries and, as the engine runs, it not only burns the glucose but also gets free energy in the process, which then gets channeled back into the batteries for later use.

Like our special car, our body's pathways provide a way for the glucose to give us free energy back *as we use it*. It's a little like getting electricity simply from the power of water flowing down a mountain. It's free and it's naturally easy to gather—so it's no wonder that it's the choice form of energy for our bodies.

Now, let's return to why it's so hard for us to keep up an exercise program, and also why it's so hard to lose weight. Glucose is always being burned—we need it in order for our brains to function. The more activity we undertake, the more glucose we burn. Although glucose is a simple sugar, it is in the carbohydrate family, which means that when we eat things such as cakes, fruits, vegetables, breads, rice, etc., they all ultimately break down (from when we start chewing them to when they are absorbed into our bloodstream) into glucose. Glucose has now entered our cells to begin the process called glycolysis which breaks glucose down and creates useable energy. It's at this point when the breakdown of glucose results in various outcomes, all of which give us energy.

Glycolysis doesn't require oxygen, so this pathway is referred to as an *anaerobic pathway*. After a series of reactions, glycolysis yields a chemical compound called pyruvate that helps prepare participation in the Krebs cycle. Pyruvate has two options, however, that it can take, reaching a kind of fork in the road. To the left is the Krebs cycle, and to the right is lactic acid formation.

In an untrained, out-of-shape body, pyruvate favors lactic acid formation. In a trained body, pyruvate favors the entrance to the Krebs cycle to be broken down even further. The key here—the goal—is to get the glucose molecules to enter the Krebs cycle to be totally broken down, because that's what yields the most free energy. In that way, we're training our bodies to fully burn glucose to its highest capacity. When we exercise, we're not training our muscles to take longer strides, finish races or complete an aerobic video—**we're training a biochemical pathway that will continue to work in the most effective, efficient manner possible for our bodies.**

Have you ever exercised with someone who could carry on a conversation while he/she runs, while you're huffing and puffing so much that you can't even get a word out? If so, you're turning glucose into lactic acid. (Remember, the first part of glycolysis is anaerobic, meaning it doesn't require oxygen.) Let's use an analogy to help visualize the process.

Start with a big jar of gumballs (see figure on opposite page). Picture another jar below the first one, where the process of getting the gumballs from the larger jar down into the second jar represents the breakdown of glucose straight through the Krebs cycle.

The two jars are connected to one another by a device with a hole in it for the gumballs to fall through. The size of the hole can be adjusted to be big or small. When we are not in shape, that hole is small, so the majority of gumballs start to stack up and eventually spill over the edge of the top jar. Every gumball that spills over the edge represents lactic acid formation, which causes our muscles to burn and ache. Those that spill over the edge *can* be brought back up and used again, however, as lactic acid can be transformed back into pyruvate and then enter the Krebs cycle at a later time.

As we exercise, the hole allowing the gumballs to enter the bottom jar grows larger, thus allowing more pyruvate to enter the Krebs cycle

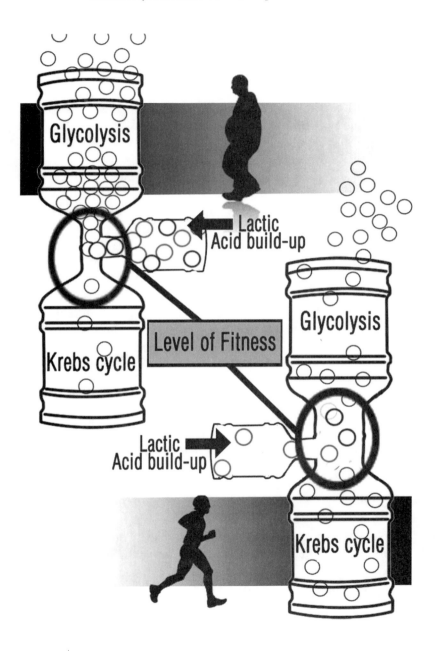

and less to enter lactic acid formation. Again, because lactic acid formation isn't an aerobic pathway, the result is that we huff and puff and feel absolutely exhausted. You see, it's not our bodies that are out of shape; it's the fact that we haven't trained certain biochemical pathways to behave the way we want them to. When we exercise, we're not only training our bodies; we're training our pathways to respond in a way that's best for our bodies.

People of different heights and weights all have the same challenges in starting a training program—and most of us give up before we allow these pathways to proceed in the proper direction! "I just can't do it," says the little (but very loud) voice in our heads. "Who am I kidding? Just quit now…think about how good it would feel to walk. Come on, I can run tomorrow… Just walk, take it easy. My knees hurt, my hips hurt, my chest and lungs hurt. Just slow down." And you thought it was only you who heard those voices! Nope, you're not alone, not by a long shot.

But when you train your pathways to respond differently, just knowing that that's what you're doing can help. Until you do train them, your body will fight you. But when you push through, you will succeed—you will have retrained your body's energetic pathways to respond in a whole new way.

Training the pathways

Start your exercise program. Keep it simple, like jogging or walking, at first. Do it long enough that you're pumping hard and breathing becomes difficult. At that point, slow down to get your breath.

The next time you exercise, increase your time by 10% with a day in between. Do it again, and then again, and keep increasing until you've achieved 10-20 increases, ultimately increasing by 100-200%. Never drop back down below where you were the prior session. When you have reached the point when you're exercising continuously anywhere from 15-30 minutes, your body is starting to pull the glucose out of storage to make it usable. Keep your heart rate up to exercise level for at least 10 minutes—or you will not have trained even the first pathway.

Exercising under 10 minutes merely creates "a bigger hole in your glucose jar"—in other words, it turns all the glucose into lactic acid. Only in well-trained individuals will lactic acid readily turn back into usable pyruvate, where it will not collect, unusable, in the body.

Prior to exercise, have absolutely NO glucose enter your system, including carb drinks. It is a falsehood that generally sedentary people need carbs prior to exercising. In fact, we have plenty of them stored in our bodies already, and taking in more right before exercising just makes it harder to train your pathways and lower your glucose levels. You do need electrolytes, but sedentary people usually have more than enough from their diets. When your exercise regimen becomes intense enough, sports drinks will be more beneficial.

> **Electrolytes,** lost through bodily secretions such as sweat, need to be maintained for bodily fluid function. **Electrolytes** are salts that conduct electricity and are found in body fluid, tissue, and blood. Examples are chloride, calcium, and magnesium. For instance, when you exercise heavily, you lose electrolytes in your sweat, particularly sodium and potassium. These electrolytes must be replaced to keep the electrolyte concentrations of your body fluids constant.
>
> Many sports drinks have sodium chloride or potassium chloride added to boost your electrolytes, but they also have sugar and flavorings to make it taste better—and keep you coming back for more.

People who are overweight have more glycogen stored, as well as more fat stored, so it will take some time to lose the weight and see results. But as long as the pathways are exercised, weight will come off. Exercising the pathways means watching one's food intake and exercising long enough with a high enough heart rate. Those who can exercise one or two hours have reached the point where they have truly trained their bodies to burn all three: the glucose, the glycogen, and the fat.

Again, energy comes from multiple places (glucose, fats, protein, alcohol, etc.), but primarily from glucose and fats. In a fit person who is exercising her pathways, when the blood glucose gets low (some people experience this in the form of lightheadedness, hypoglycemia or the shakes), glycogen or stored glucose (in the muscle and liver) kicks in. The body is trained to use the next best pathway to break down the glycogen, which can now be burned as usable fuel. Glycogen will only be burned when glucose gets depleted to some critical amount. Similarly, fats will only be burned when glycogen gets depleted to some critical amount. So, if you're not exercising long enough or with enough intensity, you could never feasibly begin to burn fat. Physiologically, it's just not possible.

A marathon runner, for example, will first deplete her glucose, and then her glycogen, until her body searches for yet another pathway. Because these athletes spend a lot of time exercising—because they're fit—they've already trained that next pathway: the one that burns fat.

Glucose, pyruvate and the Krebs cycle
When glucose burns, it turns into pyruvate, which then turns into acetyl-CoA. This process is called the glycolysis. After the complete breakdown of glucose, all the way through glycolysis, through the glycolytic pathway, and then through the Krebs cycle, the product that remains is H_2O, or water and CO_2, or carbon dioxide. H_2O is what you see on a cold morning in the Northeast, when you breathe out in the form of what looks like smoke or steam. There's water vapor there, but CO_2 also. Where does the "C" in CO_2 come from? After all, we breathed in "O_2", or oxygen. The answer is- from the glucose you ingested, from the carbohydrates. The "C" comes from the original glucose molecule that was made up of six carbon molecules. We breathe in O_2 yet we breathe out CO_2. The "C" in CO_2 actually came from the food we ate or the juice we drank!

The person who exercises regularly and stays in shape burns glucose, which goes straight through anaerobic glycolesis, where very little of it gets turned into lactic acid. That's why they can carry on a conversation while they exercise.

Using the jar and gumball analogy, if the hole through which your gumballs (your glucose) pass is small, the jar will start to fill up because only one gumball can get out at a time. You're pouring more into the jar than it can handle. Eventually, the jar will overflow. In a sedentary person, the overspill represents the formation of lactic acid without enough glucose molecules to enter glycolesis. Muscles hurt and you get tired easily.

In a well-exercised person, however, the hole from the bottom of the top jar into the bottom one is huge. The gumballs (glucose) flow in four, five, six or more at a time, so the jar on top never fills up and rarely ever spills over to form lactic acid.

That's what we mean by the pathway. The more you exercise, the more the glucose can flow and the easier exercise becomes.

When it's hard to get motivated

During my wife's pregnancy with our third child, I quit exercising. I'm not proud of it, but I put on several pounds and was so out of shape that I was shocked when I passed myself in a mirror.

I like to think I was experiencing sympathetic pregnancy symptoms because, really, I have no other excuse to offer. But it could have been any number of reasons and the end result was the same. I told myself, "Tonight I'll go running." Then that night would pass and I'd swear I'd run the next night.

It was amazing how tired I was all the time! I went to work, came home, ate dinner, watched at least an hour of TV, checked my e-mail and went straight to bed—totally exhausted. I simply couldn't muster up the strength to get out and walk, let alone run. It was one of the toughest things I've ever gone through. I have always taken care of myself, both mentally and physically, to try to stay healthy. I couldn't stand seeing myself in a mirror and, for the first time in my life, I had an idea of what so many people suffer through every day.

I decided—again—that I'd had enough! But every time I tried to get out and exercise, it was like pulling teeth. My body would give my brain excuses: *Maybe I'm coming down with the flu…Everything hurts; I can't go running right now. I'm too exhausted—I won't even be able to make it the first few steps… Just rest up, I can go tomorrow.* I had a million of them!

One evening, though, things shifted. It was about 10 p.m. and

I was checking e-mail. I glanced up at a photo above my desk of me coming through the finish line of a 15K (9.3 mile) race. I was in great shape for the race, and I remembered exactly how I felt that day—energized, positive, happy to be feeling so great physically and emotionally. I was *psyched*!

In less than a minute, I had jumped up out of my desk chair, put on running sneakers, shorts and a T-shirt and grabbed my iPod. I didn't stop to think. I went with the *feeling* behind the thoughts, which gave me all the motivation I needed. I went out, stretched and started running.

I have to be honest: the first quarter mile was nothing short of brutal. I must have told myself at least one hundred times to quit running and just walk…but I turned up the music to drown out those negative thoughts. I ran two miles that night and, sure, I was sore. My goal had been to do just one mile. But I was back on the road again and no longer felt the pull of low energy or negative thoughts and feelings about myself weighing me down.

I gave up the junk food that had somehow crept into my diet—regular "meals" that I told myself were necessary because they were easy, convenient and cheap. (Of course, now that I know they're loaded with addictive chemicals like MSG, I'm not surprised at how easy it was to become accustomed to their taste and fat content until my body craved them all the time.) And when the urge returns to be a couch potato again—which it does from time to time—I try to get through it as fast as I can.

What to do when it's not working

One of the reasons Americans have such a hard time losing weight and getting in shape (besides the usual culprits of too little sleep, poor nutrition habits, etc.) is that they've been trained to believe that their workouts should include drinking power-ades and high-carb drinks, taking supplements, etc.

We watch high-powered athletes—the tennis and cycling champions of the world—sweating and gulping down these prod-ucts on commercials. The problem is that most of us don't exercise nearly to the degree that these professional athletes do and our bodies are simply refilling the glucose we're supposedly trying to burn. Our bodies haven't learned to use the stored glucose, the glycogen, because we're constantly replenishing it. And without accessing the stored glycogen, we never get to the point where we can actually burn the fat.

Something I call "tricking your brain" can help you get started. Eat a zero-carb snack, if you feel you have to eat something. Your brain will think glucose is there because there's something in your stomach, but actually there is no glucose. You'll have satisfied your hunger urge and your body will start to pull glycogen out. The brain needs glucose or you'll pass out, but your body won't let that happen if it's been trained to start burning stored glycogen. Once that happens, your body will switch automatically to burning the fat. Then your exercise routines will be much more effective.

> **EXERCISE TIPS:** No fruit or other carbs before exercising. No sugar, even "good" sugars. No milk, no shakes. Protein shakes are okay only if there's no milk or soy (must be made with water and protein powder with zero carbs). This will satisfy urges without accompanying glucose. You may feel insistent that you need the carbs but you don't because you have them stored already. You do need electrolytes, which you can get from low carb sports drinks.

There's been a trend over the last few years to promote drinks and food related to exercising: Gatorade, Powerade, "power bars," granola bars, protein bars, and high-carb and low-carb snacks. What's the real story behind these products and do we really need them?

Gatorade (named after the Gators football team) was actually developed at the University of Florida by scientists who were investigating why athletes were hitting the wall—that is, having to quit before finishing their race. They saw that football players were hitting a similar wall; by the third and fourth quarters, they were having a tough time finishing the game.

The scientists found that when the athletes were provided electrolyte replacement drinks (full of sodium, potassium, sodium chloride, etc.) they would bounce back faster and be ready to keep playing or running or jumping sooner than before.

As we said, sweating creates a loss of electrolytes, and athletes sweat *a lot*. So adding to and maintaining their level of electrolytes is critical to maintaining the level of energy required to keep playing. However, and this is a big 'however,' glucose was also added to the drinks. In the process of studying the results, they found that adding glucose had mixed results. They determined that adding anything greater than 6-8% carbohydrates—of which glucose is one—actually *slows down* the process of gastric emptying.

For instance, orange juice has anywhere from 10-20% carbohydrates. That's why drinking it while exercising can make you sick—it slows down the emptying of your stomach into the small intestines. On the other hand, at 6-8% carbohydrates (which include high fructose corn syrup, fructose, glucose, and sucrose), the process of gastric emptying continues as it should.

In essence, it's only when blood glucose becomes depleted that you start burning stored glycogen, and it's only when the stored glycogen becomes depleted that you start burning fat. Elite athletes are performing at such a high level and intensity that they can tolerate the Gatorades and the extra carbs—not people like you and me, who might get half an hour of exercise a day. Most of us don't fall into that elite category of athletic pursuit…and that's why exercise fails.

The most common myths of exercising

The following information is based on Claudia McCoy's opinions on *The Most Common Mistakes In Exercising*. McCoy is an IFPA Certified Personal Trainer, German-licensed Physical Therapist, German-licensed Athletic Trainer, Certified Sports Conditioning Specialist, Apex certified Nutrition Coach, and Certified Distance Running Conditioning Specialist.

> *"When Dr. Scott Paton asked me to write a 'little' article about the most common mistakes that people make in their workouts, my mind took off at about 100 miles per hour. I could write a whole book just on that topic alone, I thought. I see so many people doing the same mistakes inside and outside the gym. But reaching your desired fitness goal in the least amount of time with the least amount of effort is only achievable when*

you don't get hurt in the process. That's why I'd ask that you consider the following tips to let your body burn more calories and prevent injury."

Myth #1: Cardiovascular training (or strength training) alone will enable you to reach your goals.
There are actually six components of fitness, all of which are required to help you be successful in reaching your goals in terms of overall health. They are: proper food intake; resistance training; cardio-respiratory training; flexibility; dietary support (multivitamins, protein shakes, etc); and personal assistance (some kind of personal training to learn the correct, safe and healthy way to implement all of these elements).

Myth #2: Abdominal exercises are the single best way to rid yourself of fat around the middle.
Sorry, but that's not the way the body works. The more abdominal exercises you do, the more your muscles will become cast-iron, but the cast-iron muscles will still be underneath all that fat. You won't see a washboard stomach until you rid yourself of the fat.

The best way to burn the fat deposit is endurance (cardiovascular) training in the form of at least 30 minutes of an aerobic workout in your "fat-burning-heart-rate zone." Walking, running, biking, and the elliptical bike are all forms of endurance training.

Myth #3: "No pain, no gain."
Exercise should NOT be painful. A light soreness may be okay but as soon as there is any kind of real pain, it means your body is sending out signals that you are going to hurt it. The message: evaluate your workout to see what's causing the pain. There has been no evidence whatsoever that a painful workout is required to gain muscle.

Myth #4: Injury is caused by "muscle imbalance."
Although injuries can occur anywhere and anytime, the most common injuries occur from performing repetitive movement patterns—the things we do every day of our lives. These repetitive movements cause imbalances in the musculoskeletal system that result in the overuse of some muscles and the underuse of the opposite muscles.

Left unchecked, these are often injuries that become chronic, resulting in long-term pain and dysfunction. When the imbalance is not corrected, the body is not able to function as designed. Instead of the muscles working together to perform a specified function, they work against each other, causing the body to exert more energy to perform the same task that previously the body perceived as "simple."

Chronically tight, restrictive muscles function poorly, impinging on nerves and blood vessels, and causing disorders and injuries.

THERE ARE SEVERAL EXERCISING TIPS THAT WILL HELP YOU KEEP FIT AND HEALTHY:

1. Always perform a balanced workout, training the opposite muscle groups.
2. Always stretch after each workout.
3. Target major muscle groups. When stretching, focus on calves, hamstrings, hip flexors, adductors, abdominal muscles, neck and chest.
4. Work out first. Stretch *after* your workout when muscles are warm and more receptive.
5. Don't bounce during stretching. Bouncing can cause small tears in the muscle, which leave scar tissue as the muscle heals. This, in turn, tightens the muscle even further, making you less flexible and more prone to pain.

Common injuries

Just as Claudia says, having an understanding of the biomechanics of the human body is the way to ensure exercising right. Calf strain (also known as a pulled calf muscle), for instance, is one of the most common, preventable injuries I see and is often due to ineffective stretching techniques. Once you have an understanding of the anatomy of the calf muscle, it's easy to understand why it's so susceptible to injury, and how this can be avoided by effective stretching techniques (which can be applied to other parts of the body as well.)

The calf is comprised of two muscles: the gastrocnemius and the soleus. The gastrocnemius (the larger of the two, the action of which lowers the foot, or "plantar flexes," raises the heel, and assists in bending the knee) crosses the knee joint and the ankle joint. It crosses the knee joint to attach to its origin—the point at which a muscle begins; it is that portion of the muscle that is usually closest to the torso. In this case, the gastrocnemius' origin is the lower part of the femur (thigh bone). It also crosses the ankle joint, attaching to its insertion (the portion further down the extremity, a longer distance away from the torso than the origin) at the calcaneous (heel).

The soleus doesn't cross the knee joint at all. Whereas the gastrocnemius starts above the knee, the soleus is the muscle in the calf of the leg behind the gastrocnemius muscle; it also helps plantar flex the foot. The soleus starts below the knee, where it fuses with the gastrocnemius to form a tendon, called the Achilles tendon, close to its insertion point. Although the calf muscle has two origins, it only has one insertion point where both the gastrocnemius and the soleus come together to form that common tendon *(see figure on next page)*.

Picture the leg's anatomy or straighten your own leg; when the knee is straight, that part of the calf muscle that tightens is the gastrocnemius. Try this yourself: Let your leg hang from a seated position (with your knee bent at a 90-degree angle) from a high enough chair that your foot doesn't touch the ground. Now feel your calf muscle (the muscle on the back of the lower leg just below the knee). Rub it back and forth; it should feel loose, like Jell-o.

Now straighten your knee. As you feel your calf, you'll notice

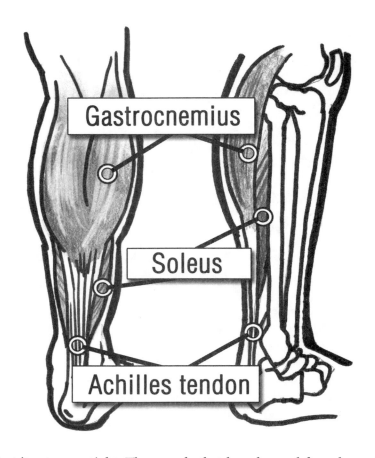

that it gets very tight. The muscle that has changed from loose to tight is the gastrocnemius muscle. The degree of tautness of the muscle that you experience will be directly related to the amount of bend in your knee. The position of the knee has no bearing on how tight the soleus is because the soleus doesn't cross the knee joint.

Lift up your foot and point your toes toward the ceiling with your knee still bent. Do you feel that tightness very deep in the calf muscle? That's the soleus muscle.

Now that you have a basic understanding of the calf musculature, think about how most people stretch their calf muscles, by leaning against a wall in a standing position with one leg farther back than the other. They push down on the heel to the back in an attempt to bring it down to the ground. The resultant "pull" is felt in the calf muscle, suggesting an effective stretch is taking place.

In reality, the only effective stretch taking place is that of the gastrocnemius muscle, not the soleus. The solution to this problem is very simple: all you have to do is bend the knee first then stretch the calf muscle. By bending the knee, you take the gastrocnemius out of the equation; it becomes lax again and the tightness recedes. This enables you to have a more effective soleus stretch.

One way to accomplish this is to interlock your fingers in front of you, palms facing inward. Put your palms just under the base of the toes with both hands connected. Pull up on your foot; you should feel a tightness down at the bottom of the lower leg, not the "calf muscle" as such, but rather in the soleus.

Another way to accomplish the same stretch is to lie prone (face down). Bend one leg and keep the other one straight. Have a partner put his hands on the sole of the foot (close to the ball of the foot) of your bent knee and "force" your toes into a position that points them down to the floor as far as they can comfortably go. Have your partner use his own body weight to slowly push down by leaning into that foot in order to stretch both muscles.

Athletic injuries, arthritis and footwear

Many problems in the extremities actually originate in the spine, not in the presenting area of complaint. If the originating problem (the spine misalignment) is ignored for too long, however, the local-ized area of complaint (the hip, knee, ankle, shoulder, elbow, or hand) will ultimately develop some type of arthritic condition in response to the imbalance and resulting abnormal wear and tear.

There are many different types of arthritis, but for our purposes we'll focus on the two most common, osteoarthritis and rheuma-toid arthritis. Medicine defines rheumatoid arthritis as arthritis that normally affects joints bilaterally (if the right joint is affected, so is the left). Osteoarthritis is normally unilateral, meaning that only one joint in a pair is usually affected (except in the case of the elderly, where joints tend to wear out bilaterally simply due to age).

Why would one knee or ankle wear out faster than the other,

given the fact that as bipeds, upright humans who walk on two legs, we use both sides to the same degree and take the same number of steps with both? As such, we might assume that both knee joints, ankle joints or hip joints would wear out evenly, but often they do not. Instead of addressing the cause of our symptoms—the arthritic condition in one knee, one ankle or one hip—we simply take course after course of painkiller, anti-inflammatory, or cortisone injection to counteract the symptoms (the pain).

Answering the bigger question of why we have the symptom on only one side in the first place can help us change the condition that has birthed the symptoms. Normally, a misalignment of the hips or the lower back has caused the center of pressure of our bodies to deviate, where we favor one side more than the other, thus adding more weight to one side of our bodies. A simple way to correct this misalignment is through chiropractic adjustment to rebalance the spine or pelvis, and is perhaps the most common way chiropractors treat abnormal wear and tear of joints in an effort to prevent arthritic changes.

Sometimes, although there is a one-sided painful condition, there is no obvious anatomic misalignment on exam or x-ray. When this happens, the first thing I look at is the patient's footwear. Believe it or not, footwear is a huge cause of other-than-anatomical misalignments. Most of us purchase our athletic shoes from sporting goods stores where the employees are not adequately trained in fitting the footwear to the person's particular anatomical and biomechanical require-ments. (Add to this the myriad of available styles of footwear that cannot possibly be good for our spines or any of our joints—high heels, flip-flops, etc.)

The simplest way to determine if your footwear is appropriate for you is to look at the bottom of your shoes. Is the wear and tear the same on both sides or is there a distinct difference between the two? If you see a noticeable difference, there is information to help you make better footwear decisions (see figure, opposite).

Shoe mechanics
In order to understand how footwear affects our body, we need to understand how the foot itself works.

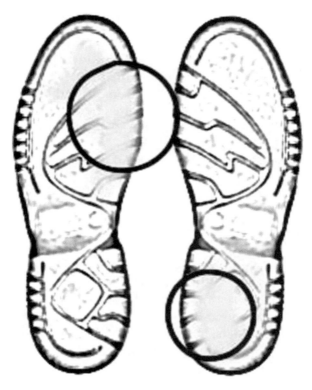

Proper foot mechanics occur when the outer corner of the heel contacts the ground first. Then, as the rest of the foot makes contact with the ground, it rolls inward (pronates). If our shoes are keeping this natural mechanical function from taking place, we will experience problems somewhere along the line. (This explanation refers to individuals without conditions such as being bow-legged or knock-kneed, to name only two. In these cases, the foot mechanics will change and do not conform to a textbook style.)

Now, let's look at the components of footwear by breaking it down into its different parts. The primary purpose of shoes is to protect your feet and prevent injury. In order to accomplish those tasks, they must fit well. Poorly fitted shoes—shoes that are too narrow, too short, or too large—can cause discomfort, injury and even permanent deformity.

WHAT TO LOOK FOR IN A SHOE

According to www.orthoinfo.aaos.org, your first consideration should be durable construction. Your feet need to be protected and comfortable. To get a good fit, the shoes should conform to the shape of your feet. Wearing shoes that are not the right fit for your feet can lead to soreness, blisters, calluses and even permanent disfigurement.

Anatomy of a shoe

The *toe box* is the area at the tip of the shoe that's rounded or pointed to varying degrees and determines the amount of space the toes will have. People with wide feet need a wider toe box; people with narrower feet need narrower ones.

The *vamp* is the upper middle part of the shoe where the laces (or sometimes Velcro) are commonly placed.

The *sole* is actually constructed of two parts, the insole and the outsole. The *insole* is inside the shoe; the *outsole* contacts the ground. Softer soles allow greater ability for the shoe to absorb shock.

The *heel*, at the bottom part of the rear of the shoe, provides elevation. An important aspect of the heel is the correlation between increased height and increased pressure on the front of the foot.

The *last* is the part of the shoe that curves in slightly near the arch of the foot to conform to the average foot shape; it enables you to tell the right shoe from the left.

The *heel counter* refers to a little plastic insert at the back of the shoe used to reinforce the heel cup of a shoe and increase support. A firm, thick heel counter cradles the heel and arch and reduces over-pronation.

The last part of the shoe to contact the ground is the inside portion near the big toe; it is the amount of plastic the manufacturer puts on the inside portion of the shoe that controls motion or the amount of *pronation*. This is called the *medial posting* of the shoe. An over-pronator, someone who aggressively rolls their feet inward as they walk, will need more plastic or another material inside to stabilize or stiffen up the shoe in an effort to prevent the over-pronation and provide support. You can tell how much posting a shoe has by simply grabbing the heel and the toe box and turning the heel one direction and the toe box in the other. The amount of flexibility/stability is the amount of control of the medial posting (*see figure below*).

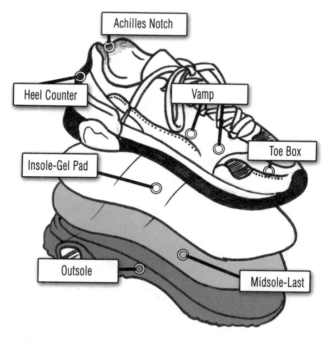

The material from which the shoe is made can affect fit and comfort. Softer materials decrease the amount of pressure on the foot; stiff materials can cause blisters.

Now that we know all the names, look inside your shoe. Shoes have insoles or cushions that are removable, and you might be surprised to learn that the insole is the most complicated part.

Inside the sole is the last; there are many different types of lasts and they differ from shoe to shoe. Lasts are either curved or straight and are further classified by their flexibility, designated by the *slip, board* or *combination lasts*. Slip lasts are better for people, like myself, who supinate, that is, walk on the outside of their shoes so they don't need a lot of structured control. Board lasts are better for people who over-pronate, whose feet roll over too much and need support and control. Some people need the combination last because their walk is somewhere between over-pronation and supination.

> **Slip Last:** An athletic shoe construction technique; also known as a California last. In a shoe with a slip last, there is no stiffening board in the insole. The result is more flexibility and less stability.

> **Board Last:** A stiffening board, commonly made of cardboard, runs the length of the shoe. Results in greater stability but lesser flexibility. Many hiking and construction boots use board lasting, whereas most running shoes use either a combination last or a slip last.

> **Combination Last:** An athletic shoe construction technique that combines the features and benefits of both a board and slip last. Combination lasted shoes have a stiffening board only in the heel area.

> **Straight or curved lasts:** Bisect the heel of your shoe (place a dot at the midpoint of the heel), and bisect the toe portion (place a dot at the midpoint of the toe), then connect both points with a straight line. If the shoe appears to be in two exact equal halves, you have a straight last. If the shoe has not been divided into two equal halves, you have a curved last. Curved lasts are better for people with high arches and straight lasts are better for those with low arches.

Your feet and exercise

Finding the proper athletic shoe is critical for a healthy workout.

If you are new to exercising and are experiencing joint pain that persists for more than 2-3 weeks, and if your spine has been examined and is in alignment, your problems likely derive from inappropriate footwear. Ignoring the situation and continuing to exercise with joint pain will only exacerbate the problem. Good walking or running shoes currently cost a minimum of $70-$160. With the right footwear, you will be less likely to suffer injury and much less likely to give up on training altogether.

To heat or ice, that is the question

Speaking of injuries, one of the most common questions I hear from patients who have been injured is: *Is it better to use heat or ice?*

The answer to that one is easy: Always use ice! Heat is often recommended because applying it feels good. Unfortunately, however, heat also pulls in more inflammation and this can extend the healing time.

One of the challenges is that a large majority of injuries are due to a secondary injury, after the first compromise of a ligament has already taken place. If a ligament has been partially torn, for example, significant inflammation causes so much pressure on the weight-bearing joints (the knee, the hip, the ankle) that a secondary, substantial injury actually occurs *after* the initial one. That's when the individual tries to compensate by limping, and that is when the most damage occurs.

When we apply ice, the infiltration of macrophages (the tiny organisms that help digest scar tissue to promote healing) will still occur; however, it simply removes the majority of the inflammation so that the secondary injury does not occur in the first place.

Recommendations

Immediately upon injury, ice for at least 30 minutes, but for as long as you want up to 90 minutes. I recommend 30-60 minutes, at least 2-3 times a day.

It's important to note that you should use water ice (ice that has been crushed so it can mold around the joint). Freezer packs are popular but can do more harm than good since the chemicals in them can freeze below 32 degrees; I've actually known people who have burned their skin in this way. If it's a foot or hand that you're icing, then use an ice water bath. Simply take a car wash bucket and put water and enough ice to make the water temperature around 55 degrees. Ice bags cannot conform around a foot or a hand, however ice water can contact every potion of the extremity.

When I was the athletic trainer at Life University, a rugby player came in after using frozen steak on his injury. The steak had stayed colder than 32 degrees for a long period of time, causing a terrible skin burn. A steak might look like a cool remedy in the movies, but this is something you should avoid.

Another question that comes up regularly is if an adjustment should take place immediately after icing. The answer here is usually no—unless icing has removed some of the swelling. In the case of considerable swelling, it can be difficult to test the joints in order to see how much the ligament has been compromised, and the last thing we want to do is strain a partially torn ligament by thrusting on it. So most chiropractors will do wait to perform a detailed examination until after the swelling has receded.

If the chiropractor has determined that the ligament has not been torn, that there is misalignment without swelling, it would then be wise to adjust to prevent further injury and to speed up the healing process.

THE HUNTING REACTION

Like many people, you may have been told at some point after an injury to ice 20 minutes on and 20 minutes off. This protocol is based on the Hunting Reaction and is often misinterpreted.

Identified in 1930, the Hunting Reaction is periodic oscillations (increasing and decreasing) in temperature levels of the skin and subcutaneous tissue after the application of ice.

When you apply ice or cold (cryotherapy), the temperature of the skin and slightly deeper than the skin will decrease; after 20 minutes, this decrease in temperature will rebound but only a fraction of the amount it went down.

People tend to misinterpret this function to

mean that after 20 minutes, the temperature will rebound to the original 99 degrees in a kind of wave cycle, continuing to go up and down every 20 minutes. For example, if the surface temperature started at 98 or 99 degrees due to inflammation, upon icing the temperature might drop to 80 degrees. The Hunting Reaction does take place in waves, but only to the point that it will rebound 1 or 2 degrees the first 20 minutes, then go back down to 80 degrees in 20 minutes, then back up to 82 degrees, etc., up and down in that way in each 20-minute cycle.

This means there is no need to ice 20 minutes on, 20 minutes off. Technically, one can ice as long as one wants, but I recommend no longer than 90 minutes at a time with a one-hour break between treatments.

Val's Story

A patient (Val) came in with a swollen knee; she was a triathlon athlete who was devastated because she had not been able to exercise for a while and, as she put it, exercise was her "*raison d'être.*" Val had already seen a friend who was an anesthesiologist. He diagnosed her with a bakers cyst and suggested surgery "to cut out the problem."

I reviewed Val's history and performed an exam. I confirmed the diagnosis of a Baker's cyst, which is essentially swelling in the back of the knee—an out-pouching of the synovial membrane, the cavity that holds the fluid in the knee.

Val's knee x-rays were generally fine; they did reveal, however, that the kneecap was deviating to one side and abnormal pressure was being applied to that knee. That was part of the problem—but the real problem, the one that couldn't be found on an x-ray, was a misaligned fibular head.

Both the fibular head and tibia (the bones below the thigh bone) were misaligned, causing abnormal wear and tear every time she ran, which had eventually caused the synovial joint to swell. The swelling ultimately caused pain and prevented her from running; it had now swelled to the point where it out-pouched through the back of the knee.

It is true that if Val had a torn ligament, she might have required surgery and should have seen an orthopedic surgeon. But an injury like that doesn't show up on any routine exam of the bigger ligaments (MCL, ACL, PCL, LCL, etc.) Some doctors will send for an MRI, but MRIs usually test negative for tears and are often "wasted" tests. (A full 50% of them are negative. If there's no tumor, arthritis, dislocation, etc. to see, the radiologists and orthopedic surgeons read them as "normal" x-rays or radiographs.) Unfortunately, with negative tests, the patient is often then sacrificed to the unlikely 'benefits' of medication.

In Val's case, there was no torn ligament. Medication had not helped the situation and cutting out the swelling (the Baker's cyst) would have accomplished only one thing—removing the symptom for the moment. If the original misalignment were not corrected, the symptom would likely return before too long and continue to get worse, preventing the patient from her enjoyment of exercise.

Val's question, "Why didn't my doctor tell me that?" is typical. Of course, there are many reasons, but ultimately they result in the same thing…the patient is not served in the best way possible.

So the *real* question becomes, "What caused the misalignment in the first place?" Could it be an imbalance in the meridians? A problem in the spine? As a chiropractor, I start with the spine—and Val's was noticeably out of alignment. It had caused her pelvis to draw up on one side, causing abnormal pressure in her knee, which resulted in the joint going out of place. This is what caused the swelling, which caused the pain, which increased the swelling…well, you get the point. The cycle had begun.

I adjusted Val's spine as well as her knee in order to restore balance and allow the healing process to begin. She came two to three times per week for treatments and was given home exercises to help stabilize the spine. Three to four weeks later, the swelling was completely gone from the back of the knee and Val was running again with no pain whatsoever.

Chiropractic is great at giving people their lives back; in this case, running was a big part of Val's life.

Val's story also illustrates two of the five essential factors for health: the importance of chiropractic care and the impact—and enjoyment—of exercise.

CHAPTER ELEVEN

NUTRITION: THE THIRD FACTOR OF HEALTH

It's a matter of self-worth

It is my sincere hope that reading this book will teach people to become more open—and part of being more open is learning to be less harsh towards our fellow human beings. We don't need to accept other peoples' behaviors or values as our own, but neither do we have to pass judgment or be critical of what we perceive to be another's shortcomings.

Judgment should be left in the hands of God, and I have found that those who disparage others are generally unhappy with themselves. Being different—whether it's size, shape, hairstyle, or sense of humor—is not a cause to degrade, condemn or belittle. Not only is that behavior a reflection on you, but a lack of compassion can also leave deep wounds on the people at the other end of your "sword." Practicing empathy or understanding, however, will only help you grow as a person.

Recently my wife and I were at Outback Steakhouse for dinner. There was a couple a short distance away who were already eating and it was quite obvious they were having a great time in each other's company. Both of them were significantly overweight.

It's no secret that obese people are easy targets for jokes and cheap stabs and, seeing them, I was reminded of how I was in high school and college. No, I wasn't overweight, but that was a time when I thought I knew everything.

I was the president of my fraternity, played on the college rugby team and dated attractive women. I thought I had it all, but I recognize now that I had very little self-esteem to go with it. We all know people like that, who spend their time making fun of others, finding people's flaws and pointing them out. It's really a matter of their own lack of self-esteem causing them to focus on what they feel are the inadequacies of others. No matter how good-looking, wealthy, or confident a person is, if they feel it necessary to debase others, it is their own self-worth that is in doubt.

So, that brings us back to the couple at Outback. As I watched them thoroughly enjoying themselves, I began to feel enjoyment myself. They were laughing, talking, and flirting—altogether unencumbered by self-consciousness. However, I couldn't help but think that at some point in time, maybe the next day, they'd run into someone who would make a hurtful comment about their weight. I thought about that because I knew it was true: I had been one of those people.

Certainly, I wasn't the only person with self-worth issues, but it is unfortunate that I won't be the last. In the meantime, it is my responsibility to be the best person I can be, which includes teaching my children to treat people with respect and a helping hand.

Health and weight

How people treat those who are overweight is a social problem; obesity itself, however, is a serious health problem not only from a medical standpoint, but also from a chiropractic one.

I've noticed that patients who are overweight have much more stress on the joints than those who are in better shape. Using a previous example, a misalignment in the spine can cause pelvic muscle imbalance, which leads to an uneven pelvis that disperses more weight through the joints of the lower extremity (hips, knees, ankles) on one side than on the other. Even in a person who is in shape and at a healthy weight, there will be abnormal wear and tear on those joints due to the uneven pelvis. Add obesity to the mix and the abnormal wear and tear turns into catastrophic degeneration of the joints at a very accelerated pace. The same goes for a much more important part of the body—the spine. And as the joints degenerate, pain sets in.

The heart also suffers due to obesity. Many overweight people have hypertension and/or high blood pressure because the heart has to work significantly harder to pump blood through their bodies. The increased blood vessel resistance, requiring the heart to pump harder, results in increased blood pressure.

Many obese patients turn to antihypertensive medications to offset high blood pressure. They are then led to believe that everything is fine when their doctor checks their blood pressure and says, "The medication is working. You're doing great!"

In reality, they are far from great.

Using synthetic methods to chemically bring down blood pressure to a medically accepted "safe level" and declaring that the person is now "fine" (i.e., healthy) is one reason why we have such sickness in this country.

The true way to become healthy is not through drugs, but by eating and living healthy. Sometimes blood pressure medications need to be used as a temporary means to keep the body from forming a life-threatening aneurism while the obese person starts an exercise program. But a doctor should never accept a quantifiable clinical test or blood test within normal limits as proof of good health.

Weight and its connection to a balanced healthcare system

Weight is a massively charged issue in our society. Unfortunately, it's all for the wrong reasons.

As a culture, we perceive weight, its loss, its gain, and its myriad of related topics all relative to how we look and how we are perceived by others. Consider the possibility of experiencing life without mirrors for a moment. How would we see ourselves differently if we were not so concerned about appearances?

What if, instead of thinking about weight primarily in terms of how attractive to others we are, we thought about it as an indicator for our level of health?

Recently, I asked Ryan Pryor, a friend and patient who owns Escapades Fitness Spa here in Florida, what he feels are the key ingredients to maintaining a healthy body, specifically related to the topic of weight and weight loss. When we first talked, I told him that I felt achieving optimum weight was a matter of self-regulation, of balancing exercise and food intake to achieve balanced health. I also said I found myself frustrated by my patients who wanted to take a diet pill to look good, without regard for their overall good health. Here is our interview:

DR. PATON: *I hate to admit it, Ryan, but it seems as if so many people want to take the easy way…take a pill or have surgery to lose weight. They're not doing it to achieve great health; they're doing it because they hate the way they look and feel pressured to look like fashion models and rock stars. They think that if they are thinner, they'll automatically be in shape. But I know they won't. I know that if they haven't exercised their cardiovascular systems and their body's cellular metabolisms, thin can also be unhealthy.*

I want to help but have trouble feeling as if I'm getting through to them. I want them to know that sometimes procedures for the grossly obese might be the answer to kick-starting the process—but that working to accomplish weight loss over time is the only way (using all five factors of health) to ensure the weight will stay off and they will be healthier in the long run.

I equate it to the prescribing of blood pressure medicine. Staying on the medicine for the rest of one's life is certainly an option, but a poor one, in my opinion, when instead the drug could be utilized temporarily until the person changes the way he or she lives in order to obviate the reason for the drug in the first place.

What's your opinion about rapid weight loss, Ryan, especially with regard to drug use or surgical procedures?

RP: As you said, Scott, I agree that in extremely obese cases there is a place for the medical facility—whether it be LAP-BAND, gastric bypass surgery [See box below] or B-12 shots—to get that initial weight loss. The "however" here is that there must be an aftercare program for people who undergo these treatments because there are always significant psychological issues going on, first in regards to how they attained their weight and, secondly, how they will respond after they have reduced that weight.

There is also the parallel medical issue of our need to actually "fire" the metabolism—change its way of functioning—for a number of reasons, in particular because that metabolism is going to change as we go through the aging process. If we don't know how our body will be changing as we go through the life cycle, and if we don't undertake appropriate steps to address these changes, we will not have the skills to be able to eat right, eat healthy, and get the appropriate exercise for our lifestyle.

So, really, it is the true lifestyle transformation that's critical. There is a place in the weight loss community, as you mentioned, for the extremely obese to get that psychological edge and possibly even get them out of some medical danger from stroke, heart attack, or any other disease that they may not have already incurred due to obesity—which, by the way, is now the number one epidemic globally.

More and more people are either dying or have diseases related to weight. In the arena of the young, we are also seeing more and more children dying before their parents in the coming years—even in the next five years—due to the diseases associated with being overweight.

DR. PATON: *One of my biggest concerns is that we know obesity is a problem in the U.S. but that problem is being seen more as a chance for profit than to help people really tackle the real problems associated with morbid obesity. How many doctors are changing their practices from primary medicine (their prior specialty) to getting some type of certification in weight loss in order to give shots and make money?*

Here's my question for you. I've recently started a nonprofit to help children in need of wheelchairs. Every year we do a 15K run called Joey's Challenge. And every year, especially if I've taken time off from regular training (like this year when my wife and I had a baby), I have to go through the paces of re-acclimating to regular exercise.

This time, just to show how difficult it can be, even for people like me who have always tried to remain in shape, I videotaped my progress. I had to start with a ¼ mile and was miserable. At a mile I heard that little voice inside me say, "Come on, just stop running. It'll feel so good to quit! Just walk now. Run again in a little bit." But I ignored it and slowly, slowly, the voice receded and I kept going. It's not easy, but I do it, knowing that the results will be worth it. Unfortunately, many people don't understand that exercise has to be a gradual process. They come to me saying, "But my joints and ankles and knees hurt too much. I just can't do it."

What do you tell these people? What makes some people unable to fight through the discomfort, unable to stop the voice? What do you, as a fitness instructor, do to keep them from not giving up so easily? What advice would you give?

RP: One of the things we do in our program is start by setting goals. When we do the goal-setting, we write a mission or a purpose statement. And when we go through that process it helps give people a sense of ownership for why they're doing this, and helps them commit to doing it.

We spend time to help them drill down to the core of why they have arrived where they are, and what their reasons are for trying to deal with that condition now. Are they here because of self-esteem issues, medical issues, to look better in clothes?

Most people do not generally come in and say, "I want to be healthier." Normally they arrive due to some kind of reaction to a situation that has become intolerable. They are in some sort of pain—physical or emotional or both. We are there to help them, to give them hope. The hope is for a longer, more fulfilled quality of life. So we have to help them internalize why they are there—not why *we* think they're there.

We know they need to be healthy. They need to come to their own realizations. "I want to be there for my kids, I want to be around for my husband, my family, I want to be a better role model, I want to think more clearly…" All these things are affected by exercise and the chemical balance of the body, and by working with them, the body can start to work for you, not against you. In turn these things will give you greater energy, have you looking better, etc.

The other thing is that we make it fun. The exercise business is not sitting you down on a piece of equipment and telling you to do it three times, fifteen repetitions. No. You have to have variety, it has to be fun, so we use different programs. It can't be boring or monotonous or people don't want to keep doing it.

Exercise doesn't always feel good and healthy foods don't always taste good to the average person. For example, in the fitness industry, only 13% of the marketplace goes to a workout facility—13% of all the consumers out there who are looking for answers.

Sixty-seven percent of these consumers go to weight loss centers, such as Jenny Craig or Weight Watchers. They want to eat and lose weight; they're still looking for the magic pill or the answer only in terms of food intake. They don't want to exercise. Don't forget, Scott, the weight loss industry is a *43-billion-dollar industry*. The fitness industry is pushing barely a 13-billion-dollar industry. You talked about doctors wanting to jump on the bandwagon? This is the future and that's why. Those people who jump into that market now are going to do very well financially.

Now, are they doing the right thing? I agree with you that they're probably not doing the right things for the right reasons. I think it's easier to give a shot, take $120 and call yourself a "weight-loss specialist." They may not have the experience, or have done the research, or have been a trainer, or focus on putting exercise and nutrition together, but that's what they do.

And then on top of all that, we need to add the critical aspect of life success coaching as well, because that's definitely something most people need.

DR. PATON: *That makes sense, Ryan. I myself have two coaches, a life coach and a business consultant, and they both help me out.*

So, what you're really telling someone like me, who can fight through that voice that tells me to stop, is that if a person can't commit to a training program on their own, they really need help.

RP: That's right. They need a program, a consultant, just like in business or in the rest of their life. And they need someone who will help prescribe what they need, hold them accountable, and help motivate them, because there have to be ongoing modifications as they go along.

Let's say there's an injury or a rehabilitation or just extensive weight gain. A 350-pound person cannot simply start running a mile a day. We need to do a lot of different things depending on the individual's needs. But the important thing is that it's a process and a lifestyle change. Goals have to be set and constantly looked at, potentially modified. We call the goals "SMaRT Goals." They're specific, measurable, achievable, and time-bound, and are associated with the larger mission the person is trying to achieve, such as maybe losing 100 pounds, but all contributing to getting the help they need.

You're absolutely right that people have a hard time staying with the program. At most any gym or fitness facility, the attrition rate is 30%. People quit after 30 days because there is no accountability, no "prescription," and people need that approach. Otherwise they need to hire a personal trainer, which is very, very expensive. We need to look at various other considerations, too. Is the program "old school"? Is it tied in with doctors, chiropractors, and other health professionals? What is the philosophy behind the program? They need a facility that will give them what they need.

DR. PATON: I always thought that if I told patients, "If I can do it, so can you," that would be motivation enough, but that's not the case at all. Because I know that when I get to the top of the hill at the first mile, it will suddenly stop hurting and I'll be able to run some more. I've experienced that so I know it will happen. But how do you personally help a client get to that point where *they* can experience it?

If I say, I want you to fast walk for the next two weeks then start jogging a half mile, then two miles, etc., most of the time the person has talked themselves out of it before they've even begun. What's your approach? What kind of tone do you use? Do you change your tone from person to person? Do you get in there like a drill sergeant?

RP: Basically, Scott, the best thing you can do is mirror your client. You've got to build a rapport and once you've done that, you kind of know the buttons to push to reach them. You can only push so far, though, if you want to maintain a professional relationship.

Sometimes you will have to take things at their pace, not yours. You're firm but fair in that you have to let them know what the consequences are…. You can say things like, "If you're going to have the McNasty sandwich, that's fine, but recognize that it's 32 grams of fat. And we're telling you that you need to maintain a 20-30 gram per day amount for us to get weight reduction, so with that sandwich you've blown it for the day." Or, "It's okay you ate that sandwich, but tell me *why* you ate it." We want to know the psyche behind their actions.

You have to work with the clients. You can't just tell them what they want to hear, because they're coming to you for hope. As soon as you allow them to call the shots, then you're on a downward slope of no results. But you can't just tell them what to do either because then you sound like a parent. You have to find a balance. You want to set *each other* up for success.

For example, if you need a chiropractor, you go to a chiropractor for his expertise. You come to me for my expertise in fitness. We let clients know that they come to us for a reason, for this experience, journey, transformation, and we're trying to help them achieve that.

Part of that is in our life coaching. This month, for instance, we're talking about "lions" or things that assassinate your motivation, get thrown at you, problems you can't avoid. We need to learn that when these lions come at us, we can take charge, kill them, put them in the ground. Our attitude is don't allow the problems to chase you and kill you; *you* become the lion chaser.

DR. PATON: *So a lot of problems aren't real?*

RP: Well, I'd say it's about reframing the problems, whatever they are perceived to be. To try to look at the reality, and work out a way to move through it and move on.

DR. PATON: *So for those people who come for an adjustment but can't hold the adjustment because they are overweight, I can't just tell them to go lose weight; it's not that simple. It's not enough to tell them to go out and jog—that if they jog and eat right they'll lose weight. Many of them can't do it, so they need help. For those of us who never really need that kind of help, we seem to figure it out ourselves, but we can't blame those who don't figure it out on our own. We need to help them get the help they need.*

And if I hear you correctly, Ryan, the reason many patients have such a hard time with sticking to any regimen is that there can be deep-seated psychological issues that prevent them from doing it. It may be a parent who always told them they couldn't do it or something else, but that deeper issue has to be approached. People need assistance to help them along.

RP: Absolutely. I couldn't agree more, Scott.

DR. PATON: *It's my hope that people reading this might begin to see the benefits of using coaches in their life—for fitness or any other area.*

TYPES OF WEIGHT LOSS PROCEDURES:

- **Weight-loss (bariatric) surgery** changes the anatomy of your digestive system to limit the amount of food you can eat and digest. The surgery aids in weight loss and lowers your risk of medical problems associated with obesity.
- **Gastric bypass** is the favored bariatric surgery in the United States. Surgeons prefer it because it's safer and has fewer complications than other available weight-loss surgeries. It can provide long-term, consistent weight loss if accompanied with ongoing behavior changes. Gastric bypass isn't for everyone with obesity, however. It's a major procedure that poses significant risks and side effects and requires permanent changes in your lifestyle. Before deciding to go forward with the surgery, it's important to understand what's involved and what lifestyle changes you must make. In large part, the success of the surgery is up to you.
- **LAP-BAND adjustable gastric banding (LAGB)** involves a surgeon using an inflatable band to partition the stomach into two parts by wrapping the band around the upper part of your stomach. Pulling it tight like a belt, the surgeon

creates a tiny channel between the two pouches. The band keeps the opening from expanding and is designed to stay in place indefinitely. It can be adjusted or surgically removed if necessary. LAGB is gaining popularity because it's a simpler procedure and has a lower complication rate when compared with more involved procedures. However, LAGB causes less weight loss and a slower rate of weight loss than does the Roux-en-Y gastric bypass. This surgery isn't recommended for people who have certain medical conditions, such as Crohn's disease, large hiatal hernias or a history of gastric ulcers.

Dieting

One of the most frustrating things I see on TV and in print ads are diet products and methods. All of the dieting methods that incorporate the importance of such things as the "glycemic index" are simply promoting easy ways to eat but not put on weight. In other words, they allow you to maintain the same sedentary lifestyle you had before, but to continue it without more weight gain.

Some diets even tell you not to eat things such as corn or carrots because of their high glycemic index. When I hear this, I cringe. At no point should a vegetable be considered inedible because it will contribute to weight gain. I suppose that if you choose to live a life in which you neglect your body and don't exercise, carrots and corn could conceivably cause weight gain—but in a life that includes exercise, the glycemic index really doesn't matter one bit.

Cholesterol: what's the truth?

In addition to weight loss drugs, diet products and gastric bypass procedures, cholesterol is a good case in point relative to medical side effects. "Doctors usually prescribe drugs to lower cholesterol. But the drugs they prescribe, called 'statins,' have dangerous side effects and, in some cases, can cause more harm than the symptom they attempt to treat" (www.loweryourcholesterolnow.com). In fact, not only is cholesterol not "bad," you can't live without it.

What is cholesterol?

Cholesterol is a wax-like, fatty substance found in all parts of the body. It's essential for good health, including that of the nervous system, skin, muscle, liver, intestines, and heart. It's a basic material used to form synapses, the pathways your nerves and brain use to communicate, and is not only indispensable for healthy hormone production but regulates the function of every cell membrane in your body.

Cholesterol can be produced naturally by the body, but is also obtained from products in the diet, found, for example, in eggs, dairy products, meat, poultry, and fish to a lesser degree. Vegetables, fruits, grains, cereals, nuts, and seeds contain no cholesterol whatsoever and fat content is not a good measure of cholesterol content.

Although all the talk about cholesterol has led us to believe that lowering cholesterol is essential (that lower is automatically better), in reality what's really important is balancing the two—the HDL, "good" cholesterol, and the LDL, "bad" cholesterol. Too much LDL can lead to atherosclerosis, angina, heart attacks and strokes, and HDL cholesterol plays more of the good guy role in collecting your system's "garbage" or waste materials—including excess LDL—and carrying it back to the liver for processing.

But the statin drugs doctors prescribe to lower cholesterol are noticeably negligent in this regard; in other words, they do nothing at all to balance our HDL:LDL ratios. Furthermore, by blocking the enzyme your liver needs to produce cholesterol, statin drugs limit the total amount your liver can create. It's not unusual, then, for the total cholesterol to fall too low, hence creating a greater risk of bleeding (hemorrhagic) strokes and death from cerebral hemorrhage.

Dr. Chris Hart, on www.loweryourcholesterolnow.com, notes that given cholesterol's status as a risk factor, we receive far more messages about taking drugs to lower it than about changing our diet to do the same.

Because we have access to what seems like an easy fix—taking a pill—even if we're encouraged to consider dietary options, we are less likely to do so. Surrounded by snack foods, fast foods, additive-laden meats and dairy products, chemical-dense food products, and sugar-heavy desserts, it's easy to see why change doesn't come naturally.

Nutritional truths

Because an approach of integrative medicine means an intelligent combination of both mainstream (Western) and alternative treatments, the emphasis of healing should be on the body's own internal healing mechanisms and systems.

Unfortunately, we don't take very good care of our bodies, and it's often only a matter of time before we are in a situation where it becomes extremely difficult to address even one factor of good health, let alone all five. The factor of nutrition, the foods we eat, is a tough one because it strikes at the heart of how we live our lives.

Everywhere we go, all around us, food has become nutritionally devoid of all the things we need to create balanced systems. Restaurants, especially fast food purveyors, use so little of substance and nutritional value that it's almost like eating nothing at all—only worse.

The four least nutritional (most nutritionally depleted) but most utilized ingredients of food in this country are: white flour, white rice, white bread and white sugar—and the value of these food items is negligible at best. However, nutrition—good nutrition—is something that we can begin to implement today just by making different choices.

Mike Adams, health advocate and author of *The Seven Laws of Nutrition* (Truth Publishing International, Ltd. 1st edition, 2006), notes that our standard diet only contributes to our incidence of chronic disease and death, as well as our rising health care costs and decreasing quality of life. The solution? Eat simple foods, focusing on unprocessed and unrefined goods.

Adams addresses an issue with white flour in particular, which is a natural insecticide; shipments often arrive laden with dead insects that have tried to eat what's in the bags. Yet, most Americans consume white flour in huge quantities, if not at every single meal. So, let's consider the question: If insects can't survive by eating white flour, how can we?

We often make the mistake of thinking that nutrition is equal to calorie intake. If we could look under all the layers of fat we Americans carry, we would see the same kind of malnutrition we see in pictures of starving people in Africa. The consumption of nutritionally depleted foods such as pancakes, white bread, candy, soft drinks, breakfast cereals, pastries and processed foods, just to name a few, is causing chronic disease in this country.

"Milk builds strong bones"…doesn't it?

Calorie intake is not the only misconception Americans suffer from. How long have we been hearing that milk is good for building strong bones and a healthy body? I've heard it my whole life—and, until recently, never questioned the validity of the statement.

Drinking milk has been an important part of being an American for as long as I can remember, and my parents made sure we always had fresh milk on the table. I only wish that I could say now that milk really is a substance worthy of its now legendary status. But the grim reality is that the only reason we believe this milk myth is because of brilliant marketing by the dairy farmers. The fact that we are sure milk is a necessity in having strong bones is literally one of the most successful forms of marketing this country has ever seen.

To criticize milk strikes at the heart of what it means to be American, and using movie stars with milk mustaches to promote the product has been a brilliant campaign, successfully making us believe that milk is indeed not only beneficial for our health, but that without it our bones would weaken along with our general health.

In reality, cow's milk has never been intended for human consumption. Other than its good taste, there has never been a reason to drink it whatsoever. The myth that cow's milk "builds strong bones" needs to be examined scientifically in order to understand the flaws inherent in that argument.

Let's start at the source. The cow gives birth to a baby calf and produces milk to feed it, just the way a human mother does. Just as a human infant needs sustenance, the baby calf needs that milk to grow and stay healthy during the first part of its life, living on it exclusively until its stomach is mature enough to handle food. Once the calf has matured, the cow's digestive system can process all the other nutrients it needs from grass and grains. So after that initial period, the calves never drink milk again. Why? Because they don't need to. *They get all of their minerals and vitamins from the grasses and grains they eat.*

So what's the difference between us and the cows?

I know it is hard to believe that we might not "need" milk throughout our lives to create strong bones. But think of it this way: When was the last time you heard of an osteoporosis epidemic among cows? When was the last time you read about adult cows breaking their hips due to weak bones? Most likely you haven't, because those problems simply don't exist—even though cows don't drink milk!

After a cow is weaned off of its mother, it never takes another sip of milk for the rest of its life. Yet it not only has enough calcium to give itself strong bones, it has enough to add to the milk that you drink! It doesn't make the calcium because calcium is an inorganic metal; it must be consumed. We need to learn from the cows that we can get our calcium from the rest of our diet.

Dr. Robert Young, a microbiologist and author of *The pH Miracle*, says the biggest misconception is that milk, being a calcium product, will give us calcium. It has been concluded now that this is not the case. Pasteurized milk actually bleaches calcium *from* our bones; it does not put calcium into them. Young says milk contains lactose, a sugar, and when this sugar is released into the bloodstream, calcium from our calcium reserves (e.g., the bones) neutralizes the acids of the sugar.

Moreover, Young says that red blood cells suffer negative effects from milk consumption; the cells stick together and become filled with bacteria and toxins. He reports that studies done in the 1980s already showed that people who drank milk each day had the weakest bones of all, while people who drank less or avoided it altogether invariably had stronger bones. In his first book, *Unlimited Power*, Anthony Robbins also cites the same research results from 1986.

Young asserts that each animal's milk is "tailored" to its species' requirements—including cows' milk, which has three to four times more protein than human milk and five to seven times the minerals, and lacks essential fatty acids of mothers' milk. Obviously, cows' milk is not made for humans.

There is every reason to believe that cow's milk in its current pasteurized form, full of antibiotics, hormones, etc., does a lot more harm than good. Fifty years ago, an average cow produced 2,000 pounds of milk per year compared with the top producers today, which give 50,000 pounds! How is this possible? With drugs, antibiotics, hormones, forced feeding, specialized breeding practices, and the latest high-tech onslaught—bovine growth hormone or BGH (used to stimulate milk production, this substance is already banned in several other countries).

In *The Milk Letter, A Message To My Patients*, Robert M. Kradjian, M.D., makes the case that as a "nation of milk drinkers," we have been led to believe—by advertisements as well as dieticians—that we *have* to get our recommended calcium intake from milk products. In light of that, you might be surprised to hear that most people today do not drink cows' milk due to taste preferences or because it makes them ill.

So who can we trust? Spokespeople for the milk industry?

Kradjian looked at over 2,700 articles from the world's scientific literature from 1988 to 1993 and summarized them as "only slightly less than horrifying." He noted that although none of the authors spoke of cows' milk as the "perfect food" we've all been lead to believe it is, they focused mainly on illnesses associated with milk, and the threat of a milk supply infected with bovine leukemia or an AIDS-like virus or contaminated with blood, pus or chemicals. Issues noted among children included allergies, infections, bedwetting, asthma, intestinal bleeding and colic; adults faced heart disease, arthritis, allergies and cancer.

Yet the Milk Industry Foundation's spokesman, Jerome Kozak, claims milk is perfectly safe. Other, perhaps less biased, observers have found the following: 38% of milk samples in ten cities were contaminated with sulfa drugs or other antibiotics (The Center for Science in the Public Interest and the *Wall Street Journal*, Dec. 29, 1989). A similar study in Washington, D.C., found a 20% contamination rate (*Nutrition Action Healthletter*, April 1990).

Robert Kradjian also informs us that in 1992, world-famous pediatrician Dr. Benjamin Spock advised avoiding milk for the first two years of life. Needless to say, many were shocked by his assertion.

To get back to my original point, antibiotics are overused—not only as drugs themselves, but also in the foods we eat and drink, including milk. This is another case where profits trump truth. My advice: Don't make the mistake of accepting advertising as gospel.

IF YOU WANT TO READ MORE, I SUGGEST:

- *Cow's Milk as a Cause of Infantile Colic Breast-Fed Infants*, Jakobsson, I., Lindberg T. (*Lancet*, 1978 Aug 26; 2(8087): 437–439).
- *Dietary Protein-Induced Colitis in Breast-Fed Infants* (*J. Pediatrics, I01: 1982: 906).
- *The Question of the Elimination of Foreign Protein in Women's Milk,* Harry H. Donnally, *The Journal of Immunology*, 1930, 19: 15-40.
- *Milk A-Z*, Robert Cohen, Argus Publishing Inc., July 2001.
- *Milk—The Deadly Poison,* Robert Cohen, Argus Publishing; 1ˢᵗ edition, November 1997.
- *Don't Drink Your Milk!: New Frightening Medical Facts About the World's Most Overrated Nutrient,* Frank A. Oski, Teach Services, 1992.
- *The Crazy Makers: How the food industry is destroying our brains and harming our children.* Tarcher Publishing, 2007.

In light of all the information, I believe we need to reevaluate how we take in our calcium requirements. The World Health Organization recommends 800 milligrams of calcium per day for American adults (the requirements are higher in this country partly because rapid calcium loss can be attributed to our lifestyles of eating meat and high-salt diets, smoking, and physical activity). Many vegetables, for example, can supply us with all the calcium we could possibly need for a healthy diet. The most healthful calcium sources are green leafy vegetables and legumes, described by the more popular term "greens and beans." Unlike dairy products, they contain antioxidants, complex carbohydrates, fiber and iron, and have little fat and no cholesterol.

"The calcium absorption from vegetables is as good or better than that of milk. Calcium absorption from milk is approximately 32%. Figures for broccoli, brussels sprouts, mustard greens, turnip greens, and kale range between 40-64%. A noteworthy exception is spinach, which contains a large amount of calcium, but in a form that is poorly absorbed. Beans (e.g., pinto beans, black-eyed peas, and navy beans) and bean products, such as tofu, are rich in calcium" (Physicians Committee for Responsible Medicine [PCRM]. Refer to the following website for more information on calcium and calcium/magnesium-rich products: www.pcrm.org).

Do I drink milk? Yes, on rare occasions, but not because it's giving me strong bones. I drink it because it tastes good. I make every effort to drink, and have my family drink, organic milk, soy milk or rice milk available at virtually any store nowadays. Organic milk comes from dairy cows that have not been injected with steroids, antibiotics, and vaccines that could cause allergies and other illnesses from a very young age.

The MSG addiction

Another significant problem in our country's food source is the proliferation of MSG, monosodium glutamate. Many of us first heard about MSG in relation to Chinese food, and most of us ate it for years in that form without thinking anything of it.

In fact, there's even a syndrome called Chinese Restaurant Syndrome (CRS), named in 1968 when a researcher identified a set of symptoms that occurred in certain people after they ate foods containing MSG. Symptoms include: a burning sensation on the back of the neck, chest, shoulders, abdomen, thighs, and forearms; pressure, tightness, or numbness in the face; chest pain; nausea and vomiting; headache; sweating; palpitations; flushing; and wheezing.

Monosodium glutamate is a flavor enhancer that has been used for nearly a century. Although the Glutamate Association states on its website that MSG does not affect metabolism, there is clear evidence from many other sources that it is not only *not* good for us, it is *addictive* and could well be one of the biggest reasons behind the massive obesity epidemic in this country.

If we look hard enough, we'll find that MSG is in almost everything we eat, from coffee to fried chicken. It hides behind more than twenty-five different labels, such as "natural flavoring," and many people are unaware of both its prevalence and potential dangers to our health. Other names for MSG include: hydrolyzed vegetable protein, Accent, and Aginomoto (a "natural meat tenderizer"), all of which can be seen on numerous product labels.

FOOD PRODUCTS THAT CONTAIN MSG

Campbell's soups, Hostess Doritos, Lays flavored potato chips, Top Ramen, Betty Crocker Hamburger Helper, Heinz canned gravy, Swanson frozen prepared meals, Kraft salad dressings (especially the "healthy, low fat" ones).

RESTAURANTS WITH MSG-LADEN FOODS

Most likely, all fast food restaurants serve foods with hydrolyzed vegetable protein or MSG, such as Burger King, McDonalds, Wendy's, and Taco Bell, but even more upscale ones like TGIF, Chili's, Applebee's and Denny's use MSG in abundance. Kentucky Fried Chicken seems to be the WORST offender: MSG was in every chicken dish, salad dressing and gravy.

John Erb, a former research assistant at the University of Waterloo in Ontario, Canada, spent years working for the government. Interested in finding out whether there was an actual chemical that caused our obesity epidemic, Erb made an amazing discovery.

While going through hundreds of scientific journals for a book he was writing called *The Slow Poisoning of America* (John Erb and Michelle T. Erb, 2003, www.spofamerica.com), he found that scientists all over the world were creating obese mice and rats to use in diet or diabetes test studies. Since no strain of rat or mouse is naturally obese, the scientists had to create them. How? By injecting them with MSG when they're born! The MSG triples the amount of insulin the pancreas creates, causing rats—and humans?—to become obese. They label these fat rodents "MSG-treated rats."

In the book, an exposé of the food additive industry, Erb said that MSG is added to food specifically for the addictive effect it has on the human body. Even the website (www.msgfactscom) sponsored by the food manufacturers lobby group supporting MSG (see box below) explains that the reason they add it to food is to make people eat more. A study of the elderly showed that people eat more foods to which MSG is added. Sure, that might benefit the elderly to some degree where loss of appetite is a concern, but where does that leave the rest of us? "Betcha can't eat just one" takes on a whole new meaning where MSG is concerned!

The MSG manufacturers themselves admit that it gets people addicted to their products, and encourages them to choose their products over others and to eat more of these products than they would if MSG weren't added.

Since its introduction into the American food supply fifty years ago, MSG has been added in larger doses to the pre-packaged meals, soups, snacks and fast foods we are tempted to eat every day. The FDA has set no limits on how much of it can be added to food, claiming it's safe to eat in any amount.

"Safe" is a curious word to use when there are literally hundreds of scientific studies with titles like these: *The Monosodium Glutamate (MSG) Obese Rat As A Model For The Study Of Exercise In Obesity* (Gobatto, CA; Mello, MA; Souza, CT; Ribeiro, IA. Res Commun Mol Pathol Pharmacol, 2002); *Adrenalectomy Abolishes The Food-induced Hypothalamic Serotonin Release In Both Normal And Monosodium Glutamate-obese Rats* (Guimaraes, RB; Telles, MM; Coelho, VB; Mori, C; Nascimento, CM; Ribeiro, Brian; *Res Bull*, Aug, 2002); *Obesity Induced By Neonatal Monosodium Glutamate Treatment In Hypertensive Rats: An Animal Model Of Multiple Risk Factors* (Iwase, M; Yamamoto, M; Iino, K; Ichikawa, K; Shinohara, N; Yoshinari, Fujishima; *Hypertens Res*, Mar. 1998); *Hypothalamic Lesion Induced By Injection Of Monosodium Glutamate In Suckling Period And Subsequent Development Of Obesity* (Tanaka, K; Shimada, M; Nakao, K; Kusunoki; *Exp Neurol*, Oct. 1978).

To read more studies like these, go to the National Library of Medicine at *www.pubmed.com* and type in the words: "MSG obese."

That's right…as early as 1978, both the medical research community and food manufacturers have known about MSG's side effects.

Many more studies mentioned in John Erb's book link MSG to diabetes, migraines, autism, ADHD and even Alzheimer's.

Here's what a friend had to say when she decided to put some of this information about MSG to the test. "When our family went out to eat, we started asking at the restaurants what menu items had MSG. Many employees, even the managers, swore they didn't use MSG. But when we asked for the ingredient list, which they grudgingly provided, sure enough MSG and hydrolyzed vegetable protein were everywhere."

The Personal Responsibility in Food Consumption Act is also known as the "Cheeseburger Bill." Though it passed the U.S. House of Representatives in March 2004 and again in October 2005, it did not receive a Senate vote either time. The proposed purpose of the act is to ban lawsuits against food producers and retailers, even if they purposely added addictive chemicals to their foods. You can read more about this bill at www.govtrack.us/congress/bill.xpd?bill=h109-554.

We like to think that we have "control" over our eating habits and that obesity is a matter of choice. But do we—and is it, really? When Erb took his book and his concerns to one of the highest government health officials in Canada, they sat in the official's office, where he said, "Sure, I know how bad MSG is; I wouldn't touch the stuff!" But this top-level government official could not be convinced to tell the public what he knew.

There are many good reasons why this kind of risk stays hidden. Big media fears legal issues from their advertisers if the public learns the truth, and the fallout for the fast food industry could mean hurt profit margins, just to name two.

What's in the food we buy?

Just as you can readily taste the difference between a slice of home-made and supermarket pie, so can you readily taste the difference between *pastured* and *industrially raised* animals. The nutritional value of "sustainably raised animals" is also superior.

According to www.sustainabletable.org, true sustainable live-stock farming must be pasture-based, with animals roaming freely in their natural environment, eating nutritious plants that are easily digestible for them. Such a set-up not only drastically improves the animals' welfare; it helps reduce environmental damage and produces more delicious and nutririous meat, eggs, and dairy.

Animals raised on open pastures move around freely and enjoy a much higher quality of life than those confined on "factory farms." On industrial farms, thousands of animals are crowded into crowded facilities, often without access to fresh air or sunlight—stressful conditions that help to spread bacteria and lead to animal illness. On such farms, animals are reguilarly treated with antibiotics.

It turns out that cattle need roughage provided by grasses and other plants, which allows them to produce saliva to neutralize acids that exist naturally in their digestive systems. On a diet of grain, a ruminant produces less saliva and more acidity in the digestive tract, which can lead to health problems including intestinal damage, dehydration, liver abscesses and death. Unfortunately, gran (corn or soybeans) is a cheap, easy way to make the cattle fat in a short amount of time, so factory farms continue this practice despite the health risks it poses for the animals.

The information below will help you make good choices for your family at the market:

- Feed-lot beef, factory-confined hogs and caged chickens create a lot of unnecessary suffering—for both animals and humans. The toxic waste problems generated from confined animals wreak havoc in both our external and internal environment. Sustainable agriculture is a way of raising food that is healthy for consumers and animals, does not harm the environment, is humane for workers and animals, provides a fair wage to the farmer, and supports and enhances rural communities.
- Quality meat producers state on their labels the percentage of pasture-derived feed; 100% grass-raised is the best but not easy to find in today's world. On the web, you can find small ranchers and farmers who sustainably raise superior foods: www.eatwellguide.org has a convenient feature that

enables you to locate growers within a 20- or 50-mile radius of your zip code. For a comprehensive statewide listing, see www.eatwild.com.

- "Case-ready" meat from a large cut-rate market is cheap, but it's also the lowest quality available. Furthermore, case-ready meat is typically altered to extend its shelf life. Pass on purchases of raw, pre-marinated meat, which may contain up to 20% of a seasoning solution...meaning that 20% of your purchase is made up of water and cheap additives. Know exactly what is in the meat you purchase.

It's best to buy meat, poultry and fish with the bones intact. Poultry and fish are better purchased with the skin intact and tend to be not only more economical but often fresher because the skin serves as a protective layer. Cooking with the bones in makes the meat, fish or poultry tastier, too. The leftover bones can also be used for soup stock.

What you need to know

These definitions should help you figure out exactly what you're getting—or not getting—when you try to shop responsibly:

- *Antibiotic-free*: As documentation is not enforced, the claim "antibiotic-free" is only as good as the producer's integrity. Purchase from a sustainable producer who raises drug-free livestock.
- *Genetic Engineering* (GE) is the process of transferring genes from one plant or animal to another. No one knows if GE food is safe to eat because the technology has not been tested properly.
- *Free-Range* implies that poultry has outdoor access but this doesn't mean that chickens actually go outside. Because it's the nature of chickens to flock together, even if there's an open door in a huge shed, the tightly packed birds tend to remain in one spot. The producer, however, is free to claim they are

"free-range" chickens simply because the coop theoretically permits outdoor access. There are operations where the birds are not as tightly packed and those birds may indeed get outside. But they're still contained in small yards without any form of plant life or insect life, and where all their food is comprised (typically) of corn, soy and supplements.

- *Sustainably raised* chickens, in contrast, roam freely and eat seeds, weeds and insects, and their diet is typically supplemented with grain. Both the flesh and eggs of these chickens are high in omega-3 fatty acids. It's an example of our ability to use words to obfuscate when the U.S. Department of Agriculture says "certified access" to the outdoors "may be sold as 'range,'" which implies but does not specify what is really required of the operator. None of the following qualifiers are included in this term: environmental quality, size of area, number of birds, or space per bird (www.upc-online.org/freerange).

- *Fresh-freezing*, to most of us, means anything below 32 degrees F but the truth is, poultry can be labeled "fresh" as long as its internal temperature does not go below 26 degrees F. A frozen-solid, "fresh" chicken at 26 degrees is called "hard-chilled" (www.upc-online.org/freerange). Ask your butcher if the chicken or turkey came in "hard-chilled." If it is, treat it as you would any previously frozen meat by using it as quickly as possible and do NOT refreeze.

- *Hormone-Free*: By federal regulations, growth hormones are prohibited in poultry and hogs. So when you read 'hormone-free' on chicken or pork labels, it is nothing but a marketing ploy. Unfortunately, hormones are permitted in fish and in 'natural' beef and lamb.

- *Natural Meat*: Meat may be termed 'natural' if, following slaughter, it is not treated with artificial additives or colorants, or its fundamental make-up has not been altered. This term does NOT refer to any foods or medicines the animal was fed or to the quality of its living conditions.

- *Organic*: Yes, we all favor organic; however, don't overlook small family farmers who can't afford expensive organic certification but who are, in fact, both sustainable and organic. Obviously, a multi-national food company's 'organic' label means less than one from a sustainable operation.
- *Pasture-raised*: A sustainably raised steer grazes in a field or pasture and, during winter months, its diet is supplemented with hay. A feed-lot animal is fed corn, farm byproducts (silage) and even animal byproducts. Ask the producer what percentage of the animal's feed came from pasture. The term 'grass-fed' is not regulated.
- *% Water Retained*: Look at the fine print on poultry labels or in meat or pork luncheon meats and you will see the percentage of your purchase that is 'added water.' More water means less actual meat, hence, the producer's profits increase. The USDA permits up to 8% added water. Just-slaughtered poultry carcasses are submerged in a chill tank to absorb as much water as possible prior to bringing them to market. You can ask your butcher to provide quality 'air-chilled' poultry (labeled accordingly); if unavailable, try to purchase poultry with 3% or less retained water.

Nutrition and supplements

The food that we eat today is not only robbed of many essential vitamins and minerals, but it is loaded with preservatives that contaminate our bodies. In order to maintain the shelf life of a particular food, it is usually stripped of many essential nutrients.

One good way to counteract this lack of nutrition is to take a good multivitamin. There are so many multivitamins to choose from that it's often difficult to know which is right for you. The multivitamins one may find at a chain grocery store are usually a colossal waste of money. A case in point was when I reviewing a lumbar x-ray of a patient, I noticed an undigested pill in his large intestine. I asked him if he'd taken any pills in the last 12 hours and he responded, "yes, my multivitamin". His was purchased at a grocery store chain. I let him know that multivitamins are rated according to how fast they dissolve in water, and he needed to do better research because the multivitamins he was taking were literally going down the toilet.

There are so many nutritional supplements available on the market from vitamins and minerals to liquids stored in what appears to be wine bottles. The bottom line is that if you know several people who are having success with the product, it's worth a try. The salesman or saleswoman may swear on their mother's grave that they have the best product, but they are usually selling the product for a commission among other things if it's a multilevel structure. I'm not suggesting that there is anything wrong with multilevel marketing, just ask for several references of current customers that could give recommendations regarding the product. If it makes you feel better then it's worth it's weight in gold.

The bottom line is that you should always get your spine checked first. If your spine is misaligned, regardless of how many vitamins you swallow or drink, you will never achieve full health. Similarly, even if your spine is aligned, you're exercising and getting enough sleep, without proper vitamins, minerals and nutrients, you can never reach your peak health.

Additives and antibiotics

I love when I hear people talking about how they only feed their families organic meats because it means they are taking the first step to a proactive approach to their health. But, for me, there is a rub. If you're adamant about giving your family only antibiotic-free, hormone-free, vaccine-free, steroid-free meats and poultry, why would you feel comfortable treating yourself and your family with antibiotics at the drop of a hat? And why would you feel so relaxed about vaccinating your children with so many vaccines? I am baffled by the disconnect that takes place in our thinking between these two obviously and profoundly connected issues.

I ask you to think about how we purposefully spend more money on products to avoid ingesting certain substances, but at the same time inject similar substances into our bodies. And I ask you to make decisions based on common sense.

Don't forget, when vaccines were discovered, we had a lot more disease *because we were living in less sanitary conditions than we are today*. Our water treatment techniques and sanitation protocols have improved to the degree that we naturally eradicated most disease in that way—not through vaccines or massive doses of antibiotics.

Considering nutrition as one of the five factors of health means considering *everything* that we put into our bodies.

A starting point

A good place to begin is through portion control. There are three main choices to promote portion control; 1) Simply take less food (you must have discipline for this one), 2) Use smaller plates, 3) drink a protein shake (flavored protein blended in water and ice) 20 minutes before your meal. The 3rd choice is probably the most realistic. It will put substance into your stomach, giving your brain a slight sense of fullness so that you don't eat as much.

CHAPTER TWELVE

SLEEP:
THE FOURTH FACTOR
OF HEALTH

On sleep

Henry David Thoreau wrote that we should wake up with nature all around us. We should wake up with the sun, the birds, the squirrels, the butterflies, because when we do, we are in harmony with the universe.

Clearly, the amount and quality of sleep we get—as well as the way in which we wake up—all contribute to the quality of our waking lives. Some experts now suggest that for every hour we stay up past midnight, we need two extra hours of sleep. For some of us, that would mean missing the morning entirely.

The universe operates in waves and cycles. When we wake up with nature, we ride those waves straight through the day and, in effect, are guided through the day without effort. When we sleep right through the morning, however, we spend the rest of the day pushing ourselves against the natural currents of the universe.

Even if you stay up late one night, it's important to make every effort to wake up early the next day to continue to be in harmony with the world around you. You may be tired, but you'll be in harmony. And part of that natural rhythm means your tiredness will motivate you to get to bed earlier the following night to set you back on course. Ignoring the cycles and waves relative to sleep is like saying you are not affected by the fact that it is sunny or raining out, light or dark. In other words, it is virtually impossible.

We have become a society that likes to say it "thrives" on very little sleep. In the past, life was indeed simpler if you consider that electricity was scarcer ("early to bed and early to rise"), we exercised more (hence, we were naturally physically tired at the end of our day), and we had less technology to keep us up and busy all day and night.

In past generations, sleep was something we took for granted—everyone expected to get a "good night's sleep" and to wake up refreshed. Nowadays, so many of us have poor sleep habits that we look to drugs to induce sleep long enough that we can function the next day. In effect, we have given sleep the short shrift—even though studies have shown time and time again that lack of sleep contributes to illness, depression, irrationality, and even obesity. The truth is, we just *think* we can get along with less sleep when we really can't. No matter how much you attempt to take care of yourself, eat right, exercise, undergo chiropractic treatment, do yoga, and/or meditate, if you don't sleep and control stress, you will be prone to disease. That's why sleep is one of the five factors of health.

Sleep: we need it!

When we sleep, we enter a state of REM (Rapid Eye Movement), during which our brains heal and become recharged. On an average night, 20-25% of an adult's total sleep is in REM, a time that is physiologically different from other phases of sleep. Most of our dreaming, at least the dreams we recall most vividly, occur during this period of REM. Interestingly, the amounts of REM sleep vary with age; a newborn baby, for example, spends more than 80% of total sleep time in this state.

It takes the body an average of 90 minutes to achieve REM. When sleep is commonly disrupted or shortened and sleep cycles do not have the chance to complete, the results can be highly disruptive to our lives and our health in general. On the positive side, it may even be possible that enhancing REM sleep can improve the next-day recall of memorization (Marshall, L; Helgadóttir, H; Mölle, M; Born, J. *Boosting Slow Oscillations During Sleep Potentiates Memory. Nature,* 444: 610-613, 2006).

Why we dream and other factors about sleep remain a mystery, but without sleep our internal clocks and bodily functions can be thrown out of sync—with potentially drastic consequences. Sleep is one of the most underrated factors of good health, which, when added to chiropractic and other alternative therapies, stress relief, exercise and nutrition, can provide the basis for healing and recharging every day—and night—of your life.

According to *S. Carpenter, Monitor On Psychology, 32, No. 9, October 2001*, lack of sleep in teens can cause cognitive and emotional problems including poor performance in school. Two of the biggest reasons recent generations have problems getting to bed on time are television and the Internet, which pull people in with an almost magnetic force. Once they've got a grip on you, they steal your time and attention and give very little back in return. When your usage begins to take a toll on your relationships, it becomes nothing less than an addiction.

Once you find a television show you like, you begin to crave sitting on the couch to watch it. Soon you're down for the count—snacks in hand. The Internet is even worse because, if television provides nothing interesting, there's motivation to turn it off, but the Internet is waiting for you 24/7. From on-line shopping to chat rooms to e-mail, all it takes is a few clicks to alleviate boredom, avoid human interaction, and often avoid responsibilities. Even when your intentions are good and you plan to just log on to check e-mail (or at least that's what you tell yourself), you can end up spending hours just tooling around.

You can tell yourself it's a harmless addiction or a compulsion, but there have been more and more reports linking Internet overuse to addictive behaviors such as gambling and illicit affairs. How can you tell if you've got a problem? If you're ignoring the needs of your family, your friends, your job—and your life—outside of the computer screen.

Isolation is one of the prime effects, and sometimes causes, of excessive time online. Interacting with *real* people is one of the primary needs of human beings. Often, previously stable relation-ships become undermined by the time online that would otherwise be spent with family members, friends, or a spouse.

On the other hand, in a society where we are becoming more

and more isolated from our communities, the Internet can seem to offer emotional attachment to online friends, even though we're sitting alone in our room. These virtual "communities," therefore, have a double-edged sword effect, not only allowing the user to escape his or her current reality, but to seek out and fulfill unmet emotional and psychological needs, which is potentially more intimate and less threatening online than in real-life relationship.

It is my belief that there is no substitute for those real-life relationships, and that avoiding them by isolating oneself can be a sure sign of an imbalanced life. Add that to the likelihood of losing sleep due to a technology addiction, and you have the recipe for 'dis'-ease in the body—a system where the life force has been compromised.

The Center for Internet Addiction Recovery is a resource for assessment and treatment of Internet addiction disorders. They can be reached at 1-800-522-3784 or www.netaddiction.com.

What is Internet Addiction? According to the Illinois Institute for Addiction Recovery at Proctor Hospital (www.addictionrecov.org), it's an impulse control disorder, similar to gambling or alcoholism, that can lead to personal and financial problems. Signs of Internet addiction include the following:

- Preoccupation with the Internet and Internet-related activities
- Requiring increased usage to achieve satisfaction
- Repeated, unsuccessful efforts to control or stop Internet use leading to restlessness, depression or irritability
- Staying online for a longer amount of time than originally planned
- Letting Internet use jeopardize significant relationships or job
- Lying to conceal the extent of Internet involvement

- Using the Internet to escape problems or relieve negative emotions

According to Maressa Hecht Orzack, director of the Computer Addiction Study Center at Harvard University's McLean Hospital, between 5 and 10% of Web surfers suffer some form of Internet dependency.

Here are my suggestions to inactivate or mitigate the hold television and/or the Internet might have in your life: Use DVRs (digital video recorders) such as TIVO to record your favorite shows and watch them in the morning while you're getting ready for your day, which gives you less time to linger in front of the TV.

Also, wake up as close to sunrise as possible. This helps align us with the universe's natural rhythm and provides enough time to incorporate some kind of meditation into our daily lives to replace the "unwinding" or "relaxing" sensations we feel we get from TV or the Internet.

Although I don't focus on the practice of meditation too much in this book, I have found it to be one of the most helpful practices I've ever undertaken. Initially, if you're doing it properly, it's common to simply fall asleep during the exercise, so make yourself comfortable and set the alarm, if necessary.

Many people often feel better about themselves and their lives—more balanced—after meditation or a good night's rest. However, most people feel even worse or more stressed after they've wasted too much time in front of the TV or computer, either from physical inactivity or compounded problems. The choice, therefore, is clear.

Not only is sleep an essential element for health in itself, it is also related to a more positive outlook and lifestyle—which brings us to the last of the five factors…

CHAPTER THIRTEEN

POSITIVE LIVING: THE FIFTH FACTOR OF HEALTH

The unhappiness factor

Some people simply radiate good will and a positive attitude regardless of their circumstances. They look at the bright side, even when things are tough. I always notice those people, and appreciate them, just the way I notice the ones who are determined to be miserable—even when life's treating them well.

What makes some people happy and some unhappy? Is it genetics or life's challenges that affect us the most? Is our happiness or unhappiness factor something with which we're born that we can do nothing about or is it a matter of choice?

Of course there are a lot of reasons people are the way they are, but I believe one in particular is that many people don't know how to be happy. Whether it's because something happened in their lives to scar them to the degree that they no longer feel capable of expressing happiness, or whether they've simply forgotten how good life can be, some people have become divorced from knowing what could really make them happy.

In our society, we have defined happiness in a way that only serves to confuse. Many of us believe that happiness is a newer, bigger house and a fancier car. Some of us are sure that having these things means we'll be happier, and are surprised to find out that all the money in the world can't buy a good marriage, loving relationships with your family, friends, and children, a satisfying existence, or good health.

We act shocked when we hear about a sports or movie star who drinks or does drugs to the point of self-destruction. When we hear these things, we say, "Well, everyone knows money can't buy happiness." The question is: Do we really believe it?

We have adopted an isolationist paradigm into our lives, which also contributes to our sense of discontent. Our cities, once hubs for communities and support, have become representative of the most alienated kinds of existence—implementing ways to avoid human contact and interaction, not ways to increase it.

Moving to the suburbs to find better lives for our children, safer places for them to play and more opportunities for growth has not created what we imagined it would. Instead, our children meet only for planned activities and retire to houses that are often very far from friends and/or relatives, where technology plays a big role in child-rearing practices. Playing in the park used to be the norm; now it's a rarity, partly due to parental fears about children's safety and partly due to our busy lives and the way we have chosen to live them.

This lack of spontaneous interaction and communal bonding leaves many of us feeling more disconnected than ever and more distanced from the possibility of living a life that truly suits us, let alone a life we would consider calling "happy."

It is my belief that many of these problems stem from a very early age, when, for whatever reason, we had to learn to *not* trust. We learned that self-sufficiency was the key to our survival—not, as we would like to believe, interdependency, love and trust. From the moment of our birth, we are separated from the primary source of love and warmth—the womb of our mothers. We are tested, prodded, stabbed and often surgically cut in the name of health and medical science.

In the '50s, the prevailing advice for new parents was, "Don't coddle. Don't hold your baby too much. Feed on a schedule." It's only recently that we are even beginning to come out of those dark days when babies were treated as entities to separate from.

Were we neglected? Did we get enough to eat? In other words, could we trust the environment to meet our needs when we needed it the most—and could we trust the people in that environment to be there when we needed them the most?

The usual words of wisdom are "Life's a jungle out there;" "You have to be out for yourself;" "Don't trust ANYONE!" On top of the now inherent fears we have about not having our needs met, not trusting that we will be cared for, and not believing that we are deserving, beliefs like these ensure that we distrust the very human need we all have to bond with other humans. As a natural outcome of this pervasive distrust, our sense of the world as a just, hopeful place diminishes in direct correlation to the lies, deceptions and injustices to which we've been subjected, leaving very little space for the kind of existence fueled on happiness.

We *can* ultimately learn to trust, but if we've been set up to expect failure from the beginning, it's not easy, especially when we come into contact with things that hurt us. With so many bad experiences out there, we 'learn' from an increasingly early age that the world is not a place of good will, we'll never find our right mate, we can never have what other people have, etc.

In the final analysis, whether we experience the ending of a relationship, a parent who falls short of a promise, an abusive situation, a coach who unloads his anger on us, or simply a sense of lack of direction, if we don't know how to come back from these circumstances with a sense of hope and faith, then our lives and our outlooks will never change. In essence, we will flounder—again and again.

The good news is that with awareness of our beginnings and awareness of our present circumstances and how we got here, we can change. We can begin to open up to the possibilities that life affords. That's what I want to talk to you about here, because I believe that if we let our guards down, even for a few moments, to let in some new information, there would be less depression and sickness in our lives—even less starvation and crime in the world.

Unhappiness causes imbalance in the system

Have you experienced a bad case of butterflies when you needed to get up and speak in front of a group? You *feel* nervous, and your body—your stomach—reacts with cramps. Have you ever experienced fear being alone in a dark place? You *feel* afraid, and your body breaks out in a sweat. Have you ever basked in the glory of a winning game of basketball or baseball? You *feel* happiness, and your body responds by laughing, jumping or even crying.

In a broader sense and over time, our bodies react to our experiences, positive or negative: to love, fear, stress, winning or losing, any and every emotion we experience. It's only natural that when we experience happiness, our bodies respond with internal signs of happiness—endorphins are released, we smile, and so on.

Awareness about not only what we put into our bodies, but about how we live and feel day to day is the only way to affect the pH levels, or the acidosis, in our bodies, and the importance of reaching a balanced pH state cannot be emphasized enough.

The happiness factor: happiness matters

I'm sure most people believe that being happy or unhappy is an emotional state, but that's only the tip of the iceberg. How we "feel" has a direct, undisputed correlation to what our bodies experience physically (and vice versa). It's been proven through study after study that the physical reactions of the body cannot be separated from the mental and emotional states of the body…they influence each other directly and powerfully. On the smallest of levels, just think about how much more energy you have when you're feeling good about something than when you feel sad.

Our bodies exist habitually in one of three possible states: basic, neutral or acidic. Of the three, the acidic condition is by far the least balanced and the worst for our overall health. Acidic conditions result in more sickness, increased healing time, and a higher risk of disease.

Currently, it is believed that over 90% of our entire population has bodies that are too acidic or are experiencing acidosis (too much acid) due to the foods we eat, the stress under which we find ourselves, and our lack of sleep and exercise.

Acidosis refers to the condition of your blood and your pH level—the actual measurement of how much acid is in the blood. Having an imbalanced pH level, particularly one that is too acidic, directly determines our quality of life. Although acidosis is not a "disease" itself, having a body imbalanced in this way makes it a virtual breeding ground for other diseases, such as cancer, osteoporosis, heart disease, high blood pressure, arthritis, obesity, diabetes, allergies, kidney stones, premature aging, and many other degenerative diseases. In fact, scientists have found that cancer actually thrives in an acidic solution and is equally as unable to survive in an alkaline environment.

Testing for pH balance is as simple as testing your urine with a piece of Litmus paper every morning (see below).

WHAT IS PH?

pH is a measure of how much acid is in the blood. pH levels are measured on a scale from 0 to 14 (0 = pure acid and 14 = pure alkaline). Our body strives to be more alkaline, about 7.3 to 7.4. A variant of as little as 2 full points towards acidity could result in instant death.

HOW TO CHECK YOUR PH LEVEL

Purchase pH strips at a pharmacy or health food store. Check your pH in the morning before eating by holding a small strip of Litmus paper under a drop of your first urine of the day. The strip will change color according to your pH level. The package will include a chart against which you can gauge your pH level and find your pH number. A normal range is considered to be 6.8-7.1 in the morning and from 7.1-7.5 throughout the day, pending you're not forming a lot of lactic acid from a recent workout. If your pH is 6.5 or below, consult a healthcare professional.

All natural foods contain both acid- and alkaline-forming elements. In some foods, acid-forming elements dominate; in others, alkaline-forming elements do. Acid-forming foods include animal proteins, cooked oils, alcohol, pasteurized dairy, caffeine, refined/processed grains and carbohydrates. Environmental factors that induce acid include: smog, radiation, pesticides, chemical preservatives, food dye, and additives. Exercise—the right amount, too much, or too little—can create a more acidic or more alkaline state in our bodies.

Sometimes, for example, people are so concerned about losing weight that they exercise several hours a day. When they do not see the results they want quickly, they become frustrated and stressed, a state that can also create too much lactic acid in the body. That's why I always advocate regular but moderate exercise.

Our thoughts, emotions and stress levels are linked directly to the varying levels of acidosis and alkalinity in our blood. Worry, anger, fear and distrust are all strong factors for creating an imbalance of acidosis, especially when we experience these sensations on a regular basis. The body's reaction to this kind of emotional stress is a powerful statement for incorporating deep breathing techniques and/or various stress-management techniques to offset some of life's challenging moments and maintain a balanced system.

Begin to change things

So you're beginning to realize the importance of staying positive but you're probably wondering where to begin. First, make a list of all of your problems and then look at them for ten minutes per day, but never, never before you go to bed. Focus the full 10 minutes on action plans to alleviate those problems but then don't look at them or think about them again that day.

Second, take a look at the people you are associating with. Without our realizing it, they can be directly related to our moods. There are destroyers and there are builders. Builders choose to see the good in people and they're not interested in talking about another person's misfortunes behind their backs. (A piece of advice is if you're talking to someone who's discussing another person's shortfalls in a way that doesn't help that person, you better believe that the minute you're not around, the discussion will shift to *you* and your shortfalls.) People like these are destroyers who will suck the positive energy out of you like a pick-pocketing thief.

Builders don't dwell on the negatives; they smile a lot and regularly give congratulations or praise. They emit positive energy and help you get positive hormones flowing, knowing that if you want to see the good in people, you must respect them first and give everyone a chance before passing judgment.

Understand one massive, important thing: If someone pulls a fast one on you by losing your trust, taking your money, etc., you must let it go. Keeping it inside will only raise your acidity and further ruin your life. They may think that they got one over on you, but they didn't trick anybody. The Universe has a way of taking care of earthly garbage. It's not your job, so just move on. One big piece of advice; don't ever go to bed thinking about a person who upset you. If you do go to bed thinking about them and stressing out, they own you. You let them own you.

On qi, the flow of energy, vibrations, and the universe

Things we take for granted—in fact, ignore—actually have huge repercussions in all aspects of our lives. For example, we've all heard that every human being, every animal, plant, and atom in the entire universe vibrates, although we feel none of those vibrations. We know that the Earth moves around the Sun, and that we are moving, too, because we're on Earth, though we don't feel any movement at all.

Scientists have also proven that on a subatomic level, everything in the universe is made up of energy. And because health is the balanced, harmonious flow of life's energy (*innate* or *qi*, as previously discussed), imbalances in this flow due to unhealthy habits and/or negative emotions and stress lead to illness.

Throughout history, the idea of universal energy pervading all nature has been held by mystics and in religious practices, but it is only very recently that Western scientists have joined in this belief. Referred to in the Indian spiritual tradition as *prana*, by the Chinese as *qi*, and exemplified in Christian religious paintings as halos of light surrounding religious figures, this vibratory energy has now found acceptance by scientists with the aid of technological research. This research includes holographic patterning, Kirlian photography, scanning, and other ways to observe the very real human energy field.

For example, tuning forks are vibratory tools. Remember seeing your piano teacher tune the piano with one? Now, they are being used as simple, inexpensive tests to determine hearing loss or if a stress fracture is present. According to www.healthatoz.com, increased pain when the fork is placed on a bone can mean that a stress fracture is likely.

Tuning forks come in different frequencies, are measured in hertz, and vibrate at a rapid speed. If you put a strobe light on a tuning fork, you can actually see the metal bend back and forth as it makes its high-pitched sound. If you take two tuning forks vibrating at the *exact* same frequencies, put one on one side of the room (propped up so that the part that vibrates is suspended) and then tap it, the one on the other side of the room will begin to vibrate also. It's as if the two tuning forks are communicating through vibratory frequencies.

Human beings vibrate as well on an atomic level that we cannot perceive; however, we vibrate through an extremely large spectrum of multiple frequencies every single day. Here are a few examples: Have you ever been on a date and somehow knew that you were about to get dumped? You felt vibrations and your body interpreted those vibrations by giving you that sick feeling in your stomach. Have you ever had someone try to hide it or surprise you, but you knew good news was coming…you could feel it? What you felt were vibrations, which the other person couldn't possibly hide.

This last example shows that we must be extremely careful because, even when we think we're hiding some emotion, we're not. So after you've had a bad day, let it go, let the universe sort it out. Please don't take it home because those negative vibrations will emit from you and infect your spouse and your children.

Therapies that incorporate vibrational or energy modalities include Reiki, which, according to www.reiki.org, focuses on inviting "stuck energy" to move. Reiki stimulates the body to heal and instigates a purification process that can lead to greater vitality. If one's "life force energy" or *qi* is low, then they are more likely to get sick or feel stress, whereas a balanced energy system is the best defense against disease.

Humans tend to dismiss connections of a vibratory nature, but in fact they take place all the time, and we rely on them and react to them as purveyors of information. Connections between human beings based on attraction or mutual dislike, for example, are often vibratory in nature. We may have no reason to actively like or dislike another person, but simply "feel" a particular way. When we sometimes "know" that we're about to receive good or bad news just from the tone of someone's voice, that "tone" is simply another way to refer to "vibration."

In the same way, using vibration as a tool can be useful in contributing to the healing process. Chaos, on the other hand, conflicts with healing and alignment. Negative vibrations inhibit the healing process.

My patients often tell me that our office is very "positive" and I'm convinced that such an environment helps with healing. After years of seeing the results, I know that positive mental attitude contributes as much as any other modality to the healing process.

Likewise, a negative attitude continuously projected inward and outward (to the world in general and/or to particular people in particular) will make it almost impossible to create an environment in which a person will be successfully healed. As we all know, being around negative people brings us down, too—in vibratory terms, our higher level of vibration will lower in response to their lower vibrations and we will find ourselves feeling worse for that connection.

MY PERSONAL PROMISE

I believe that when you give to the Universe, the Universe gives back to you, so I try to send out as many positive vibes as I can every day. There are days that don't go as well as I hoped, however, and sometimes I know I've been pulled down by my own negativity. So, quite a while ago, I made a promise to myself. When days like this happen, I pull out my checkbook, find a sick or less fortunate child in need through a charity of my choice and write out a check—on the spot—for a donation.

Not only am I happy to help a child in need, I know that regardless of my previous negative thoughts, I'll be more than gratified by the giving I've done.

I've learned to turn around many of my negative

thoughts since then, but I still donate—just because
I want to.

The thing about vibrations is that, while we can change them as we change our outlooks, we can't fake them. So it doesn't pay to try to lead a double life, acting a certain way around colleagues and in your community then going home and becoming a different person with your family. As Don Miguel Ruiz says, "Be inscrutable with your word" (*The Four Agreements: A Practical Guide to Personal Freedom, A Toltec Wisdom Book,* Don Miguel Ruiz, Amber-Allen Publishing, 2001). Keeping a level head and integrity will mean fewer frustrations and less reason to come home and take out your stress on your family.

In essence, balancing your inner self with your outer self only contributes to your ability to promote self-healing and alignment— not only alignment in a physical sense, such as alignment of the spine, but alignment of your thoughts and actions toward a defined goal.

On communication

I'm proud to say that aside from a few rare occurrences, my wife and I communicate very well. I've designed a rule about communication that works so well for us that I would recommend it to everyone: When something makes you mad, it's easy to spontaneously become unglued and let out your frustrations on an unsuspecting spouse. It's not fair and it's poor communication. What I try to practice is waiting twenty-four hours when something rubs me the wrong way.

It's not that I suppress it, but I think about it, sleep on it, and if it's still on my mind, bothering me the next day, then I tactfully bring it up to my wife. If it's so important that I haven't been able to let it go, I make the time to talk about it, explaining that I thought I'd get over it but I haven't. We end up discussing the issue and always feel better for it. There's no animosity when we talk because we're both after the same thing: a better relationship with the best communication possible—all of which contributes to a positive attitude.

The twenty-four-hour waiting period makes sense because the hormones, the epinephrine, that are pumping through your body when you initially feel that anger or disappointment has abated, at least somewhat. At that point, you can speak more sanely. Lots of times, after a day has passed, you're not even fazed by the thing that was bothering you in the first place. You can just let go and move on, realizing it was never that important.

The 80/20 rule

Have you heard of the Pareto principle? Also known as the "80/20 Rule," this principle states that, for many events, 80% of the effects result from 20% of the causes.

It was in 1941 that Joseph Juran, business manager and expert on quality management, suggested the principle and named it after Italian economist Vilfredo Pareto, who observed that 80% of income in Italy went to 20% of the population. It quickly became a common rule of thumb in business that 80% of sales come from 20% of the clients.

The reason I raise this topic now is because we can apply this principle to many relatively more mundane matters: for example, we wear 20% of our favored clothes about 80% of the time, or spend 80% of our time with 20% of our acquaintances, etc.

I have extrapolated this theory to reflect a certain trend I see in the world: 80% of the population is made up of followers; the other 20% are leaders. When I use the term "leaders," I don't necessarily mean a political figure, business owner or high-ranking military official. Leaders in this case are people who don't always maintain the status quo and they're not bashful when it comes to speaking up when they feel something's not right.

Neither category is inherently good or bad, and neither is genetically predestined. In fact, any one of us can shift from one to the other by choice. And that's where it gets interesting: You can be a great follower, but you won't necessarily have opened your mind yet to the many possibilities for self-improvement, awareness, furthering your knowledge, and improving your health. When you choose to become a leader, however, you start to consider your options. You put your foot down or question authority. You ask questions to empower yourself and get the answers you need to make sound decisions for yourself and your family's well-being.

It's not about holding a powerful or prominent position; it's about you as a human being, as an individual responsible for the results in your life. It's about recognizing that if you fall into the 80% category of "followers," you're not particularly concerned about the "whys." You simply do as you're told or make decisions based on what is expected of you. You may not care why certain things are the way they are—and you may not have much of a desire to allow change to occur. This may be where you are currently or where you were in the past but either way, when you decide to change that paradigm for living, you immediately become part of the 20%.

And there's no going back.

As a 20-percenter, you empower yourself, whether purchasing a new home or making health and medical decisions. You take a firm stand by listening to many opinions, trying new paths, considering alternatives before making decisions or before doing what comes easiest or what you're told to do. Leaders don't let people push them around; they think every decision through carefully.

When you're in the 20%, the only people you should "follow" are those making strides to achieve the same goals you are—the ones open to possibilities, not closed to what they do not yet know or understand. Here is my advice on becoming a 20-percenter:

- Never take advice from someone with a negative opinion of something he has never tried. As a self-proclaimed 20-percenter, I've seen a lot of results of bad surgeries come through my office, but I know that doesn't give me the right to disparage all orthopedic surgeons.
- Make every attempt NOT to get bent out of shape. When you feel yourself becoming agitated, try not to "let your tongue fly." It's easy to give in to an instinct to fight back in a heated moment when someone offends you or says something negative about you, a family member, a close friend—or even your politics. The 80% group will lose control and say or do things they wouldn't normally do,

embarrassing themselves in the process. The 20% group is quite the opposite. When I say leaders put their foot down and choose not to get walked on, sometimes that means simply walking away.

· Avoid negativity at all costs. When I'm with a person or a group of people in a private setting and they talk negatively about someone not currently present, I simply walk away. I don't trust anyone who says negative things behind a person's back or who turns a person's downfalls into public gossip. If I hear it, I literally raise my eyebrows, smile and say, "Excuse me, I need to make a call" or leave to use the restroom. Rarely will anyone the 20% group gossip about another person; that's one way I know I'm talking to a leader. Please understand I'm not saying that every person who falls into the follower category isn't nice or gossips about others; I'm saying that you're more likely to find these people in the 80%.

The 80% group largely consists of those who can't say "no." They have trouble committing to a task and sticking with it; they say they're going to make a lifestyle change, improve their exercise regimen and their diet, yet they never do. Regarding health, it's easy for the 20% to make educated decisions and stick to them.

I have patients in both groups. When I make dietary or exercise recommendations, some apply them immediately. They may ask why I'm making those recommendations or what they can expect in certain timeframes after they apply those regimens, but that's what makes them leaders. The other 80% would say, "Thanks for the recommendations," then never apply them. I can explain the five factors of health to a patient and a leader will take advantage of and apply the information; a follower usually will not.

Some patients who fall into the 80% will show up to an appointment looking exhausted. I'll ask, "How's your diet? Are you getting enough sleep?" Like clockwork, they'll say, "I'm not getting enough sleep because I'm stressed out at work." I ask how many hours they're working and they respond with some ungodly number. Those types of people can't follow the five factors of health because they're not willing to make a career change or a lifestyle change.

I can tell a patient is transitioning from the 80% group to the 20% when they come in smiling, looking forward to a career change, a move or a life-altering decision they made. Inside, I'm cheering. Outside, I smile and say, "Congratulations for doing something you need and want." Essentially, that 20% has the positive attitude that will ultimately improve their lives.

The faith and health connection

A lot happens in the universe that can't be explained. Scientists make it their life's work to find proof of all sorts of theories, to explain that which has so far gone unexplained/unexplored. For me, I have come to realize that taking a leap of faith can sometimes be much more important.

It's like that first jump off a diving platform. You may be afraid and shaking, but when you land in the water, you cheer and wave your hands around as if you just won the World Series because you realize how much fun it was. You wonder why you got so worked up and nervous in the first place. There are two reasons: 1) we're leaping (literally, in this case) into the unknown to experience something we've never experienced before; 2) we've all made bad decisions in the past and paid the price. Therefore, one of the most common reactions is to create in our minds a negative outcome for something that hasn't even happened yet.

Many of our fears and problems exist only in our minds; if we thought about them differently, we might not be afraid. In fact, we might not have them at all. Sometimes we focus on what we perceive to be problems to the degree that we actually *will* them to occur. Or we worry so much that we prevent ourselves from pursuing what would be the right direction.

One of my biggest "universal taps on the shoulder" occurred when I decided to go to chiropractic college. At that time, I was an environmental chemist for Westinghouse and had already been accepted into the University of South Florida's College of Public Health for a Master's degree in Environmental Chemistry, which Westinghouse would pay for since I was furthering my education in a related field. I was just out of college, had a nice vehicle, was doing well. I wasn't crazy about some of the traveling requirements of my job, but it was a great position that I felt lucky to have.

Back then I didn't attend church very regularly, though my belief in God and respect for His work was a constant in my life. I tried my best to do nice things for other people just on principle. I didn't spend much time thinking about the universe or how it attracted good things into my life. In fact, my priorities were pretty clear: work, money, success.

When I received my first adjustment and knew at the most fundamental level that something had changed, that I was supposed to—needed to—be a chiropractor, I was not prepared. The fear that engulfed me was enormous and my instinct told me to run as fast as I could from what I was feeling. The voice inside me said loudly, "No, no, you can't do that. You've got a good job, stability. Don't make a bad decision." The universe, on the other hand, would not let me off that easily. It was not just nudging me, it was screaming: "DO IT! DO IT!!"

It was one of the toughest decisions of my life to leave the confines of my safety net, anticipating no full-time income for the next three to four years, and finish school with six figures of debt.

Talk about blind faith!

The bottom line is that I did it and, every day, I know it was the right thing to do.

Staying with what's comfortable and safe, from a job we're not satisfied with to an unhealthy relationship, only puts off the inevitable—more unhappiness.

Living a positive life

Again, I need to be honest: I hesitated about adding this section to my book. But there was really no way I could have written it with the integrity it deserves—and the reader deserves—without including how I feel about the subject of having the faith to continue living a life of positivity, even when things get tough.

I haven't always lived the healthiest or most responsible life. It's hard to admit, but it's true and I want you to know. It's been a long road, packed with struggle and joy alike. But I have arrived at a place where I can honestly say that without my belief in a greater power,

I would not be here today—with a beautiful wife, an amazing family, and a career in which I can actually experience the benefits of healing every day. Here's the short version of what happened to me. I hope that in the retelling, it helps you also:

For a long time, I felt the best way to manage my life was to have total control. I worked very hard at having that control because I believed without it, I'd be miserable. What really ended up happening was that I became so rigid in my need for control that I'd be miserable whenever something didn't go my way. In fact, I got so used to controlling things and *making* things go my way that I lost all ability to bend or change direction when they didn't.

Naturally, I'm not suggesting that we abdicate all responsibility for making things happen or directing their course, but I am saying that complete control of one's self and environment may not necessarily be the best way to live a happy, healthy life.

Back in the summer of 1995, I had just graduated from the University of South Florida with a chemistry degree and was feeling relatively out of control because I hadn't found a job that I wanted yet. I finally took a job working in the Tommy Hilfiger section of Dillard's department store. I used to say to myself every day, "Imagine that…a college grad working in the men's department of a clothing store for only a bit more than minimum wage."

Even though I knew jobs were scarce, I was very self-conscious about what I perceived to be the lack of a high-level enough position. I berated myself daily for what I felt were my failings, and felt angry about what life wasn't offering me.

During the first couple of months, I tried to focus on being happy to be out of school without tremendous responsibility, away from tests and the pressure of performing. But I was still dismayed by my lack of income and prestige, and the fact that I wasn't challenged or working to my full potential was grating on my self-esteem. Sure enough, before long I began to resent my position altogether and wish I'd never taken it on.

One day a customer came along who told me she was a medical sales representative. She went on and on about what a good match I'd be for that kind of job and even said I had a "look" that would be great for medical sales. It turned out she was the regional sales director for Tampa and the surrounding areas at a large pharmaceutical company.

I didn't need much prodding. Finally, my big break! I'd heard how medical sales was a glamorous life with a handsome income. So, after speaking to the woman a few more times, I said I'd go for a job interview she offered to set up in Atlanta. They were willing to fly me out and provide transportation…how could I say no?

The day came and I put on the one suit I owned and my cheap shoes then left for the airport early in the morning. I'd never had any interview coaching so I was nervous but confident. After all, I was smart, wasn't I? I deserved a break, didn't I?

When I arrived in Atlanta, my stomach was in knots and I didn't know how to handle my attack of nerves. I met with several of the company officers in detailed interviews and by the end of the afternoon, my mind and body were exhausted from the stress. By the time the last interviews were underway, things got worse, fast. I wasn't "*feeling* it" anymore; I'd lost the excitement and was ready for it to be over.

When I left, my hopes had plummeted and I'd already decided the position was lost.

Within a few weeks, I received a letter stating that I was right—no job. Boy, was I bummed out! Back then there was no "life is a journey" philosophy for me, no "*gee, that's too bad…but what's next?*" kind of reaction. There were only two ways for me to see things: success or failure. And there were no small failures, no scrimmage game losses, just big "Super Bowl loss" failures. I had no faith that things would improve or my true calling would ultimately reveal itself.

I could not foresee that in a short time, my life would be transformed by a simple experience. I did not know that getting my spine adjusted for the treatment of a back problem would ultimately change my life. I did not question the "whys" of my situation or how I could change the outcome.

Why have I told you all this? Since my life has turned a corner when I made the decision to become a chiropractor, I have been more and more appreciative of how important it is to be open to life's possibilities, especially when we feel trapped by our circumstances.

Being in a healing profession, I know now that there can be no real healing, no real connection with the people who come to me for help, if I am not connected with the universe, my inner self and my Source. My patients come with all sorts of problems. They feel downtrodden and depressed, sick and afraid, full of whatever it is that made them that way—whether it is anger, anxiety or issues left unresolved for sometimes an entire lifetime. It's my responsibility to help open them up to the unlimited potential their lives have to offer through understanding and chiropractic care.

I learned many lessons while studying to become a chiropractor and the biggest challenge arose when I began to see that conventional "healing" techniques quite frankly were not what I expected. It didn't take long for me to discover that the new techniques and tools I was being taught were only a portion—a small portion—of the therapies available.

Sure, I learned conventional medicine. I studied and took tests and kept my mind focused on the end game. But it's only when I began to really look at why some patients healed and some didn't, why some treatments worked and others didn't, and why the same could be said for my own life, my own health and my own state of mind, that I began to see a deeper and more meaningful approach.

I knew I needed to really look at a human being in a holistic way—and see all the positive potential they possessed—in order to accomplish true healing results.

On karma

It's amazing to me that the kinder, more honest and open I have become, the better my life—and the life of everyone I touch—has become. We've all heard of *karma*, right?

According to Hinduism and Buddhism, karma is the action seen as bringing upon oneself inevitable results, good or bad. It is the cosmic principle in which each person is rewarded or punished according to his deeds. Karma reminds us that God wants us to live our lives without feeling compelled to point out the flaws in other people, to avoid excessive criticism, and to use praise often and in a loving manner. When we remind ourselves to consider the karmic principle, life becomes better for everyone.

But here's what really happens. Not only do we go about our daily lives without considering the consequences to others, we actually avoid looking at the consequences to ourselves!

We live in a world with so much anxiety and stress that we get to the point where we need to depend on medications to tranquilize us enough to bear it. We depend on medications to perpetuate a level of denial that keeps us going and enables us to live lives often devoid of meaning or full of pain. We take drugs to handle the potential anxiety that hits us when or if we consider trying to do things in a new or different way. Transformation or challenging the status quo is not always an easy road to travel, especially when so many of us feel we're walking that road alone, against the flow, and against the power of the "norm."

It's often the case that because we have so much anxiety and turn to medications to relieve us of it that we never manage to look directly at what caused it in the first place. Sure, we might know our job is tough (on a good day) or is killing us (on a not-so-good day), or that our marriage is crumbling, or that the abuse we suffered as a child has been swept under the rug. But it's easier to deal only with the symptoms of these ever-present problems than to air them out for review. Popping a pill in our culture has become as easy as taking a drink, both well-established methods for avoiding the present reality, and often promoting a lack of emotional connection with those around us.

We carry around our burdens, not really looking at them, until our negative lifestyles cause us to feel that a fifty-pound rock is chained to our neck. Over time, that rock gets heavier and heavier, never letting us be, never letting us rest, and certainly never letting us flourish to our true capacity.

Of course I remember the days when I had a huge rock around my neck, feeling stressed, miserable and guilty about many aspects of my life and certain that I would never get a second chance. I had already made it through chiropractic school and should have been thrilled at my successes, but I was still trapped by a feeling of not being good enough or never being able to have what I want.

I'll tell you another story, and we'll see how positive actions play into all of this.

Another story

One day, a short time after I opened my current practice, I was supposed to meet a friend at the local Cracker Barrel—only because he was buying, mind you...I couldn't afford to buy myself breakfast.

I was pretty miserable that day, most days really, and didn't really want to go but, hey, a meal's a meal, right?

My friend met me with his wife's cousin and, after we all sat down and ordered, we sat back to wait. My friend's wife's cousin (we'll call him Mike) had been keeping up a steady flow of talk, but I hadn't really been listening, focused as I was on the choices of a hot breakfast.

Now, though, as I listened more closely to Mike's chatter, I couldn't help feeling that I really didn't want to be there. He was laughing at and making fun of everyone he could, moving from one person to the next, pointing out perceived flaws in the people around us. He wasn't particularly discriminating: an overweight woman received as much ridicule as a guy with a mullet. As Mike continued to poke fun at anyone who entered his line of vision, I began to feel sick to my stomach. I felt sicker and sicker with each passing minute. In fact, I didn't know if I would be able to eat my long-awaited meal when it came.

I tried to change the subject, all the while asking myself why Mike's pronouncements were bothering me so much. He seemed a pretty good sort for the most part, smiling and congenial. Why was I feeling this urge to punch him in the face?

I decided to give Mike the benefit of the doubt: He was probably insecure, had problems of his own, had no idea how his lack of sensitivity was coming across to other people. Were any—or all—of these excuses true? I had no idea. But I knew right then and there that he was dragging me down. Literally. I began slipping down in my chair, embarrassed to be with someone so negative and insensitive, and embarrassed that I wasn't saying anything to stop him.

The sad thing to admit is that had I not been in a mental lull, I may have joined in and poked fun as well, but God has unique ways of teaching us humility, and sometimes those lessons come when we're at the bottom of a barrel. I had left a good practice in Georgia, where I was used to my time being occupied with treating patients, to start a new one in Florida, where patients weren't exactly knocking down my door. Today's breakfast happened to be at around the two-month point after opening my practice, and things were definitely still slow.

I didn't know it then, but it was a perfect time for my humility lesson.

When the food arrived and I didn't have to converse, I thought about how being miserable (or insecure or just plain mean) was like a cancer, and how a cancerous attitude had effects and caused reactions that went far beyond the moment.

I thought about how if you're feeling miserable, there's no way you're in a good position to give advice on being happy, to motivate someone or to contribute to their well-being. Then I thought about how being in this miserable state would affect the body. I knew that misery felt acidic, felt bad, felt wrong. And I knew from all my training that on a physical level, producing too much acid was a sure way to throw the body from a neutral state into one of potential illness.

As I was contemplating how my own misery might be impacting my health and state of being, I looked up from my plate to notice a heavyset woman at the next table. In big letters on her T-shirt was the single word "Me-ma." "Me-ma" is what my son Tyler called my mother when he was too young to say "Grandma"—in fact he calls her that to this very day. As I looked at the woman, she smiled at me, a very warm, friendly smile. I knew I was also smiling from the memory of what "Me-ma" meant to me. The woman was there with a man I assumed was her husband and he also flashed me a smile and gave a friendly nod.

At that moment, my friend and Mike got up to go to the restroom, but I stayed behind. I had the overwhelming urge to connect with these two people at the next table but I didn't want to do it while Mike was there. As soon as they left, I opened the conversation by saying I couldn't help but notice the woman's T-shirt and explaining what it meant to me. The woman was delighted and we talked for a few minutes about where she got the shirt (in a small town in Tennessee) and how she had never found another one like it.

As the conversation was coming to a close and my friends came back to the table, I shook the couple's hands and thanked them. I couldn't believe how talking with them had made me feel so much lighter, so much less miserable. Here were two smiling, positive people who had changed my entire perspective.

In a few minutes, we got up to leave and my friend went to the cashier to pay the bill. It was then that I saw the woman from the next table coming over to me, a paper bag in her hands. She walked right up to me and said, "Here, this is for you." In my surprise, I didn't notice that she was no longer wearing the same shirt. She'd actually purchased a new one from Cracker Barrel to put on so that she could give me a gift of her "Me-ma" T-shirt! Even my friends were impressed with the sheer, unbridled nature of her generosity.

I can still remember the rest of my day and how I felt like a new man. I must have called ten people to share the story and let them know how special that woman was and how she made me feel. The rigor of starting my practice ceased to bother me because that woman's graciousness made it seem irrelevant—or at least more hopeful.

So, to the lady in the "Me-ma" shirt, *thank you*. Your actions showed just how much a positive attitude can impact your own life and well-being, as well as the lives of others. You are part of the inspiration for my writing this book.

CHAPTER FOURTEEN

THE IRRATIONAL SIDE OF MEDICINE

Knowing what's best for you

Now that we've taken a close look at the five factors of true health and seen how relatively easy they are to accomplish, it's not difficult to imagine the direction your health will take if you buy into the false information and fear-mongering that spreads throughout society—and is often initiated by those in the medical community.

Perhaps one of the most difficult aspects of having a chiropractic practice is hearing from a patient that their family physician or pediatrician has expressed annoyance (or dismay) about their seeing a chiropractor. This story is representative of those I often hear:

Today a woman I'd been treating came to the office with her son for help with his chronic torticollis or "wry neck" (a condition in which the head is tilted toward one side, and the chin is elevated and turned toward the opposite side), as well as for a couple of other health issues such as ADHD and regular nosebleeds.

This young man, "Jack," had been treated with several medications for his nosebleeds and for the Attention Deficit without improvement. A thorough examination and x-rays showed there were several misalignments in his spine, which I addressed with a series of gentle spinal adjustments. Soon Jack began to feel great, with no more complaints about neck pain, a complete cessation of his nosebleeds, and an increase in his ability to be more focused and alert.

The exam and x-rays had also identified one other potential problem, early signs of scoliosis. This mild case was directly related to a leg length inequality where one leg was slightly shorter than the other, causing Jack's hip to drop on that side. (There are other, rare causes of scoliosis, which cannot be corrected and should not be attempted.) Jack's case was treatable with a small lift in his shoe that would act to even out his pelvis, thus promoting the correction of the scoliosis.

Shortly after my work with Jack (based on years of research on the subject of scoliosis and leg lengths done for my Master's thesis), his mother brought him back to the pediatrician for a revisit. She commented to the doctor how much his nosebleeds and neck pain had improved but was unprepared for the tongue-lashing she then received. The pediatrician verbally attacked her for taking her son to a chiropractor. Although she argued on behalf of the chiropractic treatment, saying it was working when nothing else had, the pediatrician refused to listen and criticized chiropractic for being much too "invasive."

When Jack's mother went on to tell him which leg I had indicated required the lift, he argued that it was the wrong side, showing her with an "eyeballed" measurement. He suggested in no uncertain terms that she take Jack to an orthopedic surgeon for further evaluation. When she asked what the orthopedic surgeon would or could do, he responded that they would saw the leg in two then separate the halves by the same amount of inequality between the two legs. They would then cast the leg to immobilize the separated bones and let more bone grow in.

Jack's mother returned to me in a state of anxiety. Afraid she was doing the wrong thing, she felt rattled by her doctor's reaction and fearful about her son's health.

I was flabbergasted. The pediatrician had not noted the scoliosis, but based on an unreliable eyeballed measurement was confident enough to tell her that chiropractic was too invasive and suggest she have her son's leg cut in two. In my estimation, a doctor like that is allowing his opinion, his ego, and any misinformation guiding him to come before his patient's health and best interests.

If a patient is experiencing improvement in his/her symptoms from non-invasive therapy, another healthcare professional should be supportive of the results. If the patient experiences no sign of improvement over a period of time, the medical doctor has every right to suggest trying other avenues.

Dealing with a closed-minded doctor

If you've experienced the benefits of chiropractic care or know someone who has, you may have found yourself promoting those benefits to others. In some instances, your remarks may have been accepted and respected by receptive people interested in knowing more about chiropractic. Some may even share their own experiences or their family's experiences with chiropractic care.

Unfortunately, things may drastically change if you bring the word "chiropractic" up in some medical offices. Granted, if you've been hurt or treated improperly by a chiropractor, your doctor has every right to protect you and direct you toward alternative forms of care. However, if you have had a positive experience with chiropractic and it's helped changed your life for the better, your medical doctor should be pleased that you are improving, period.

To this day, many medical physicians allow their own egos and negative opinions to permeate into the last place it should: the patient treatment room. If you ever find yourself in this precarious position, take what he or she says with a grain of salt, then walk out and find a new doctor who's willing to put your health and well-being in front of their prejudices.

Doctors should be obligated to treat from a positive, supportive angle. If a form of healthcare is making you feel better and improving your quality of life, shouldn't s/he be happy for you as a patient and as a person? Do you really want to trust your health to someone who denigrates other professions and professionals? Discrimination of any kind has no business infecting the confines of a treatment room, in which a person is searching for better health and answers about what's best for them.

Discrimination is not selective. It is a horrible, despicable practice that should be frowned upon whether it's toward another person's skin color, heritage, religious belief, or belief in healthcare. Discrimination from medical doctors, whether toward chiropractors, acupuncturists, or naturopaths, is unjustified. If their opinions are because they feel chiropractic is unsafe, they should think again—and do more research!

I, and nearly every chiropractor I know, hold ten times as much malpractice insurance as does virtually any medical doctor (in Florida), including surgeons—and we don't perform any type of surgery whatsoever. Surprisingly, even though we have ten times as much coverage, we pay one-tenth the amount that medical doctors pay (for substantially less coverage)! Malpractice rates are directly related to damages that physicians inflict on a patient. So if chiropractors can afford to hold ten times the coverage as most medical doctors, what does that say about the safety of chiropractic? It's extremely safe! The myth that chiropractic is dangerous to patients is completely shattered to pieces by malpractice rates alone, let alone hundreds of thousands of patients' experiences.

The bottom line is if your intention is to get healthy, stay far away from people who bring prejudices and closed-mindedness into a treatment room, because good health will be the last thing you'll find in that office.

"Natural" and "alternative" remedies: detecting the truth

It's unfortunate that so many potentially life-saving and life-enhancing methods and treatments have been disparaged by the Western medical community for so many years. Promoting these remedies as "kooky" at best and irrelevant or dangerous at worst has done nothing to help patients learn to help themselves.

Again, it's important to ask the right questions, be our own health detectives: Why does Western medicine tend to be so against other types of treatments, even those that have been practiced in different parts of the world for thousands of years? Why are we so focused on illness instead of wellness?

To get to the bottom of these issues, we have to again ask: Who benefits from this disparagement? And the answer is unequivocally: Insurance companies, Big Pharma and many physicians. After all, prescribing drugs has become the first and foremost method of so-called "treatment" in this country.

For example, the FDA has been attempting to oversee and regulate sales of all vitamins and supplements. Some might say that it's to regulate our safety, but I believe it's simply to control a manner of wellness and healthcare that has previously not been under its auspices. With companies free to promote their own alternative treatments, drug companies see the potential loss of patients to these other avenues, which ultimately leads to less income for Big Pharma.

It's no coincidence either that doctors are jumping on board with supplement promotions now that the market has grown considerably. Those same doctors who blatantly condemned the use of supplements now suggest vitamin C regularly to their patients to boost the immune system. What changed? Their ability to make money from their recommendations.

The article "FDA Seeks Stricter Regulations for Alternative Medicines" in *Insight Wellness News* (April 2007, *www.anxiety-and-depression-solutions.com*) explains that if the medical establishment can't profit from these alternative treatments, then stricter regulations will see that they remain less available. According to the author, under a new guidance document up for review, the FDA is proposing stricter regulations on herbs, vitamins, vegetable juices and even "devices" such as massage oils, massage rocks and acupuncture needles. The National Center for Complementary and Alternative Medicine, a branch of the National Institutes of Health, defines complementary and alternative medicines basically as anything that is "distinctly different" than the practices of conventional Western medicine This includes acupuncture, massage therapy and aromatherapy. The FDA has produced a document stating that the yearly visits to CAM practitioners outnumbers those to primary care physicians.

"Guidance" or "rule"?

The FDA is claiming that the regulations they would like to institute would be utilized for "guidance" purposes, to determine exactly which CAM items should be further regulated. But the CAM community is in disagreement, believing that it is a blatant attempt to control the use of those items in America under the guise of "looking out for the peoples' welfare."

In the view of the FDA, they should be regulating any item that can be used to treat or prevent disease. This means that if someone claims their breakfast bar helps cure cancer, the FDA has the right to regulate that bar as a *drug*. It also means that if someone is using hot stones as part of their massage therapy treatment, those stones will be regulated as *medical devices*.

When I was attending chiropractic college, and even long before that, many medical doctors were pushing antibiotics so hard that, at the drop of a hat, they would prescribe them for almost any symptom, even a slight tickle in the throat. Chiropractors were vehemently against this form of therapy, arguing that staying healthy is by far the best road, and to do this by practicing what I call the five factors of health (which includes taking appropriate vitamins and supplements as part of balanced nutrition).

The medical community scoffed at chiropractors, arguing that since we are prohibited from prescribing medicines, we compensated by promoting vitamins. Did they really believe that was our motivation…or was it a stance based on feelings of superiority and an unwillingness to consider the health benefits of treatments other than medication? We will never know their intentions. But the truth is that, like me, most chiropractors use what they know to help people avoid treating symptoms with medication, and have made the choice to practice healing in that way. Even being labeled "quacks" didn't deter those of us who believe in our cause.

Chiropractors continue to urge their patients to not be so quick to turn to antibiotics, but rather to let their body fight off the infection on its own. The medical community insisted—and many still insist—that vaccines, antibiotics and drug therapies are the answer. But now we are seeing that the opposite is true. Not only are we creating our own diseases through the chemicals in food and in the air, but drugs created to treat these diseases often cause more problems than they correct.

Needless to say, over-prescription has ultimately created a dangerous environment for us all, and points to the fact that we need to change our thinking toward staying healthy, so that we have less of a need to treat illness. Extreme measures become necessary for those of us who have not taken care of our bodies so that by the time we go for help, we find ourselves needing to react quickly, no longer able to afford the luxury of making the kinds of lifestyle decisions we might otherwise have chosen to make.

Although chiropractic and acupuncture don't technically "treat" or "cure" disease, they encourage the body to heal itself by becoming balanced. And stories abound by people who have chosen to pursue therapies that the medical establishment eschews—and who have not only survived but thrived.

Diagnosis: death

Given that some in the medical establishment want to eliminate competition and put profits before patients' health, I find myself once again obligated to comment on a particular aspect of the medical profession that concerns me: accepting a death sentence from a physician.

By now, readers should all have some idea of how much a person's emotional and mental states factor into how the body will function. Once the body has succumbed to an imbalance, which has manifested in an illness such as cancer, it might well be true that the imbalance is harder to adjust or correct. But to most of us, the statement that we are beyond help can be devastating and is likely to contribute to our own debilitation.

Who can say just how much a positive attitude and belief system will contribute to our health and recovery? Simply put, you help create your own future. This idea is new to many and anathema to some. But it is becoming more mainstream as increasing numbers of people tap into their own intuitive processes in order to find more satisfying answers to their questions about life, prosperity, health and well-being.

Think of all the survivors out there—people who have been told there is little or no chance of survival. I've seen it with my own eyes many times. As a volunteer athletic trainer (as a member of the medical staff) at a number of cancer walks, I have spoken with people who were diagnosed with all kinds of cancer: prostate, ovarian, uterine and others. Most had one thing in common: they had survived far longer than their doctors had predicted—and each was part of a proud, exuberant group.

The important question to me is not only why our society is so concerned with insisting on "death dates" in the first place, but why these particular people, these survivors, have lived on past the time-frame given to them by doctors.

Let's return to my earlier discussion about the relationship between negativity and acidity in the body, and their consequent relationship to illness. Because we know that high levels of acidity contribute to less of an ability to heal and stay healthy, we also know that this state of being makes us much more susceptible for illnesses of all kinds. Clearly, a life of negativity (especially in combination with bad nutritional habits, lack of regular sleep and little to no exercise) is a combination for certain (or near certain) ill health.

Among other things that occur with continued negativity are: clogging of the arteries, headaches, fatigue and depression. Your body has less ability to heal when you're not in a positive state of mind, and to be positive, you must feel good. There is no drug that will make you feel good without any side effects.

The best way to start feeling good is through chiropractic, acupuncture, meditation, proper diet, proper rest, proper exercise, proper hydration and positive thinking. With the right factors as the foundation, everything else, specifically good health, falls right into place.

What this discussion brings to the forefront is the tremendous need we have in this country to focus on wellness as opposed to illness. Even the idea of 'prevention' establishes the idea that we must continually be fighting against disease, and that puts ideas of illness in our heads and hearts before we've even begun.

We need to start thinking about doing everything we can to align our physical selves with the vibration of our "higher selves." I know that probably sounds strange to most people but think of it like this: If I say, "I'm going to beat this illness," then the idea of illness continues to be firmly entrenched in my thought processes. If I say, "Everything I do contributes to my physical well-being," I'm establishing that good health is my primary focus—*not* illness.

We have been taught to think in certain ways that contribute to the way we live and consider our health. We can teach ourselves to think differently if we so choose. But we have to first be aware of the mindsets we hold and be willing to change them in order to see positive results—despite what some doctors tell us.

Keep in mind those meridians and energetic pathways that run through the body. According to www.easternhealingcenter.com, allowing our *qi* to flow freely along the meridians keeps us free from illness; blocking the *qi* brings pain. This idead underscores important Chinese medicinal principles according to thousands of years of wisdom and the same is true for negative—blocked—thought processes, which can also create both physical and emotional pain.

Pessimistic thoughts are like sending out arrows of negativity that attract only more of the same, piercing your body both physically and emotionally. Like the scare tactics and death sentences passed out by the medical community at large, they do not contribute in any way to our overall well-being!

CHAPTER FIFTEEN

THE BODY DETECTIVE

Searching for answers

Healing the human body is a topic of vast opportunity and knowledge, and the more we open ourselves to possibilities for different approaches to healing, the more likely we are to experience their benefits.

As I have said, my own education in this area of achieving health started the very first time I experienced the benefits of chiropractic care for my sore back. In those days I was virtually uninterested in any form of care that strayed even the slightest from the norm—the norm being Western medicine, drug therapies and the like. But when the norm stops working, we search for what will.

Since then, being open to every possible avenue for healing, as opposed to only the ones I believed were worthy of my attention, has changed the way I see my patients, my life and my health. In essence, I've become a Body Detective.

Although "modern" medicine has always, for the most part, regarded the human body as a physical and chemical system that becomes ill when any chemical imbalance in it occurs (and has, therefore, treated this imbalance with external chemical substances), it's clear now without a shadow of a doubt that treating the chemical/physical body as a separate entity, one which exists apart from our spiritual, emotional, and mental parts, makes absolutely no sense at all. Looking at the impact of all aspects of our lives on our health is the only smart thing to do.

Biomechanical and kinetic chains

To probe yet another layer deeper in our search for answers about how our bodies are affected by what we do, and to understand how everything in our bodies, minds and spirits is connected, we can look at the system of body mechanics, called biomechanics.

Biomechanics is the study of the mechanics of a living body, especially of the forces exerted by muscles and gravity on the skeletal structure. A physical examination, for example, which includes biomechanical screening, will identify related imbalances in posture, alignment, strength, and flexibility.

For instance, if the problem area is an aching knee, we might first begin by testing the range of motion of the foot because the foot is always the first and last thing to hit the ground throughout the day. The manner in which the foot hits the ground is the beginning of a biomechanical chain reaction—a sequence of events—that will affect the rest of the body.

You've heard the phrase: "You're only as strong as your weakest link." This is indeed a true statement from a physiological perspective because our bodies are connected in more ways than you might imagine. Long-standing problems often can be referred back to imbalances elsewhere, particularly (as indicated previously) in the spine or hips.

Within this biomechanical chain of events is another one, called the *kinetic chain*, which pertains to, causes, or is characterized by all motion in the body. Again, the reason it's referred to as a "chain" is because all movement is related to some degree, on some level. Pain in the feet might be due to problems in your calves or knees. Pain in the knees may be due to problems in your hips. Tight calves can lead to problems in your knees, hips, and lower back, which, in turn, could lead to problems in your upper back, shoulder, neck and even head. Learning what the correct cause of the problem is, and treating the cause—not the symptoms—is clearly the only truly effective way to enact healing.

Naturally acute injuries (injuries that have just happened and are the result of an outside force or trauma) do of course occur, but generally speaking, more of the injuries I see are old problems that were never addressed, or addressed correctly. Examples include:

- The patient is compensating with one part of his/her body because of another injury, such as when more weight is placed on one side to take pressure off the other (as with a "bad" or injured leg).
- The patient has muscular imbalances, which lead to over- or under-compensation of other muscles, as in the case of problems in the shoulder where some muscles are overdeveloped and others are left weak. This sets up another kind of compensation process that can lead to injury.
- The patient has scar tissue (or "adhesions") that has developed due to previous injury. Extensive scar tissue can limit range of motion and cause resultant problems in the joints.
- The patient has been using "movement patterns" inappropriately. This happens when we play golf or swing a tennis racquet or paddle a kayak on a regular basis and always do it incorrectly. In time, not only will your ability to do the particular sport suffer, but imbalances in strength and flexibility will ultimately occur, as well as inevitable pain and overcompensation patterns.

Let's use, as an example, a problem that causes the pelvis to draw up on one side and cause more weight to be placed on the other side; that, in turn, may present as a symptom in the ankle joint. Presenting with a sore ankle may result in going to a medical doctor to have the ankle joint injected, but the real problem has not been addressed and the ancillary problems will inevitably continue (possibly after a brief hiatus, in response to the drug received).

Chiropractors refer to this kind of misguided treatment as

"chasing the symptom." That's why chiropractic emphasizes the wisdom of looking carefully at the kinetic chain before making a diagnosis.

Let's examine the "kinetic" part of the kinetic chain to understand what is behind the linkage of events. A baseball pitcher, for example, stands on the mound before he throws a pitch, gathering his energy. You could say he has a great deal of potential—stored—energy at his disposal in that moment. As he takes that first step backwards and raises his arms above his head, he's building up a lot of kinetic—moving—energy. He lifts his leg, and as it reaches a high point, he has built up the rest of his potential energy to use during that pitch.

At this time, he will begin to unload all the stored energy he has amassed. He takes that step toward home plate and twists his body toward the batter during the windup. Then, in almost a whipping motion, he flings his body forward, letting the arm drag behind then pulling it forward. That's a perfect illustration of the kinetic chain in action from lower to upper extremity.

Now, let's say that our pitcher has a dysfunction in his hip. When he goes to make the pitch, he doesn't quite kick as high as usual, which means he's amassing less kinetic energy. As he takes the step forward, it may be shorter; without question, he will lose velocity on his pitch.

The catcher will recognize it; the pitcher will recognize it. The catcher may ask why he's pitching so slowly and the pitcher's ego may take a hit. His response may be to try to make up for that slow velocity by overusing another joint, usually the shoulder, elbow or wrist. Although he may increase the velocity, by overusing one or all of those joints, he is likely to cause an overuse injury. (Most pitchers call it being "armsy" when they're throwing more with their arms than with their whole body.)

So, because our pitcher's original hip imbalance remained unnoticed (it quite possibly manifested no symptoms at the time except for a decreased range of motion), he overcompensates with his shoulder joint (or another joint), and a week later goes to the doctor with pain in that joint.

Although most chiropractors don't have a pitcher's mound in

our offices, in a case like this we ask the patient to do what are called *functional movements* to uncover imbalances in the kinetic chain.

One way to do this is to have the patient lie face down and lift each leg, one at a time, as high as possible. Then the patient turns over and repeats the leg lifts, one at a time, with a straight knee. We check ankles, knees, hips, shoulders and spine, looking for the cause. In some cases, we find the presenting joint of pain is indeed the problem, but most of the time, the pain has been referred from another area altogether.

The athletic detective: athlete physicals

Now that we are on the subject of sports, I would like to address the myth that chiropractors do not have the expertise be the on site physicians for sporting competitions. My knowledge as well as other sports chiropractors regarding sports injuries has helped many athletes, both young and old. Our very conservative way of practicing healthcare helps deal with two of the most overlooked injuries; potential heart conditions that may lead to sudden death and concussion.

I occasionally read about young athletes, usually under the age of thirty, who die suddenly, sometimes in a city marathon, sometimes on a high school football field. Being an athletic trainer, I have become aware that some of these incidences may have been prevented—not by exams, but by recognizing family history, and then applying certain measures to offset genetics.

Especially in the world of athletics, there are factors that can either make diagnosing an injury—or the source of a problem—easier or more difficult. One of the things that makes it particularly challenging is the fact that examinations take place in an office—not on a track, on the baseball field, or in the gym, where the athlete is actually in the midst of experiencing all the bodily events related to the physical activity h/she is undertaking.

My background as a certified athletic trainer has given me the opportunity to learn a great deal about the heart. I would like to share some of this information with the reader; if I can help save even one life, it will be worth the effort.

Pre-participation physical examinations (PPEs) were intended to identify medical conditions in advance, in order to affect safe and effective participation in organized sports. But, for the very reason stated above, they are not always effective at uncovering potential problems. An exam in an air-conditioned room, on a comfortable padded table, in a quiet atmosphere will not be conclusive for all conditions in which athletes find themselves. By their very nature, sports activities bring with them potential heat exhaustion, racing hearts, heat stroke, dehydration, etc.

Males outnumber females 10:1 for sudden death, and the majority of these cases are due to a condition called hypertrophic cardiomyopathy. Hypertrophic cardiomyopathy is when the muscle inside the heart enlarges in an asymmetric way—one wall enlarges more than the other walls. When the muscles enlarge (become hypertrophic), they take up the space—or the volume—that the blood used to occupy, and when that happens, the heart is pumping less blood than it used to.

Hypertrophic cardiomyopathy is consistently a silent killer because it is not detectable by auscultation (when doctors listen with stethoscopes) or usually on electrocardiograms or EKGs. The only way to identify this condition is by having an ultrasound of the heart (echocardiogram or ECG).

A similar condition is called left ventricular hypertrophy, in which there is more of a symmetrical thickening of the heart muscle in the left ventricle. This condition is usually sports- related, due to a rapid increase in activity, and often self-resolving; however, it is still life-threatening if undiagnosed by a cardiologist. The cardiologist can recommend certain activities from which the athlete should refrain to avoid this kind of risk.

If you look at the causes of sudden death in athletes under the age of 35, approximately 50% are due to hypertrophic cardiomyopathy and approximately 20% to left ventricular hypertrophy. Coronary artery disease comprises around 10% in this group and other common anomalies comprise the remaining 20%. Interestingly, cases of hypertrophic cardiomyopathy in those over 35 drop to approximately 5%. However, coronary artery disease, makes up about 10% of the under 35-year-old group, jumps to 80% over 35.

Warning signs of sudden death in athletes

If you or anyone you know has any of the characteristics below and has not had a stress test with ECG, automatic referral to either a pediatric or adult cardiologist for a stress test, EKG and especially an ECG is recommended:

- Family member who died suddenly under the age of 50
- History of fainting while exercising
- Dizziness or light-headedness during exercise
- History of heart palpitations
- Heart murmur (sometimes acceptable; athlete may be perfectly fine)
- Family members who are very tall and have long fingers as well (a condition called Marfan's Syndrome)

This is one of those cases in which, even if your insurance will not cover the ECG, it's well worth the outlay of cash. I recommend these tests for anyone active in sports to ensure that the heart walls are normal, and for anyone with any of the above characteristics who plans to enter into an exercise program for the first time to get checked by a cardiologist beforehand. Because these problems are rarely identified in a standard physical exam, in many cases more thorough, specific testing is the only way to identify and avoid a potentially deadly event.

Concussion

In the United States, we are challenged by the fact that concussions have no commonly accepted grading standards. Research and statistics have no validity relative to this subject.

REALsports on HBO did a show on this topic for which they interviewed individuals from both the medical and athletic sides. The medical perspective is that concussion is unlikely to cause future problems, and they cite a vast array of research to support their argument. The players, on the other hand, insist that concussion can cause potential permanent brain injury and cite research to support their claims. So although there is valid, peer-reviewed scientific research available, it is both confusing and conflicting.

Early in this book, I wrote about how research and its use of statistics can drastically skew results. If I didn't personally have prior knowledge about that, I would never have believed how "scientific research" could be so contradictory. In this case, I have seen enough proof that I know that multiple concussions *absolutely can* cause permanent brain damage. Unfortunately, however, the verdict on long-term consequences of multiple concussions couldn't be more polarized and without indisputable research, we face the typical conundrum for treatment options—or even lawsuits to pay for medical bills.

Concussions are generally graded as level 1, 2 or 3. The Cantu, the Colorado Medical Society and the AAN (American Academy of Neurology) systems vary slightly, yet are all commonly accepted. Some of the grading systems claim that when an athlete is knocked unconscious, the concussion should be considered a 2; however, other systems disagree, claiming it constitutes a 3. The bottom line is that the team physician or athletic trainer has the freedom to apply the grade of whatever system he/she sees fit, sometimes whichever one will legally ensure protection from liability when allowing an athlete to return to play.

Each level or grade has a different "return-to-play" protocol. An athlete with a grade 1 concussion is the first to be able to return to play then with a grade 2 then 3. Obviously, the tendency for the team physician, especially in college or professional sports, where a lot of money is at stake, is to use the most liberal grading system because it will allow the athlete to get back on the field, court or ice the fastest.

When it comes to children, I, as an athletic trainer, use the most conservative grading system in order to protect their well-being. Athletic trainers receive significant training in identification and management of concussion. There is more information available every year, and the NATA (National Athletic Trainers Association) does a great job of providing that information at license renewal symposia.

After a concussion

Every once in a while, a parent will tell me his/her child had a "grade 1" concussion—that the child did not black out, nor did they have any light headedness or memory loss. They tell me their pediatrician's advice was to "just watch him through the night and wake him up every hour on the hour to make sure he's okay."

I shake my head and think, "I wish your pediatrician would go to an NATA symposium." More current information shows that that advice is the last thing you want to follow. A grade 1 concussion is a mild "brain bruise," so to speak. It rarely manifests into anything more significant and normally shows little or no symptoms other than tenderness when the skull is touched (if the skull contacted anything hard at the site of impact), or a short-lived headache. For such cases, we need undisturbed sleep to recharge since during sleep is when our brain and body heal themselves.

In the REM state, we are most deeply asleep so it is then that the brain recharges, allowing us to feel well rested the next day. It takes approximately 50-90 minutes to enter REM sleep, and we usually enter it multiple times throughout the night. If we continuously wake the child up every hour, h/she will not be able to reach REM even once. When deep sleep is averted, the brain never gets truly rested, thus the child wakes up with many secondary, unrelated symptoms due to a poor night's sleep. These secondary symptoms sometimes lead to expensive and unnecessary diagnostic tests.

When I am serving as an athletic trainer at a sporting event and witness a head injury that I grade a 1, I take the time to explain a few things to the child's parent or guardian. Some of the problem signs, indicators of a more serious injury, of which parents should be aware are:

- Uneven pupil sizes
- Non-reactive or slow-to-react pupils to light (i.e., pupils appear to be larger than they should be when light is shined in the eyes)
- Poor anterograde recall (test for short-term memory), such as recalling three simple words ten minutes after being told them

- Nausea, vomiting or vertigo, slurred speech, inability to focus attention or delayed motor or verbal responses

If any of these symptoms is present, the child needs to be examined by a physician in a hospital setting immediately.

However, if you have been told by a trained and licensed medical professional that your son or daughter had a grade 1 or <1 concussion and doesn't show any of the above signs or symptoms, let him/her sleep through the night. If you feel compelled to check on the child throughout the night, that's okay, as long as you don't wake them—but *you'll* be the one suffering in the morning from lack of sleep!

Concussion grading should only be done by a trained and licensed medical professional, and the information I tell parents only relates to a grade 1 concussion. In the case of a grade 2, I recommend significant and detailed medical examinations before the child leaves the field to determine if there is a need for further diagnostic testing. In the rarer case of a grade 3 concussion, an automatic hospital transport by EMS is the correct thing to do.

Medical referrals

I have to say it again: medicine is a good thing. If my patients need referral to a specialist of any kind, I am the first person to help them get there.

All I ask is that you take as good care of yourself as possible and that you act as your own health detective by exploring all your options.

CHAPTER SIXTEEN

SUCCESS STORIES

What works

It's important to discuss the ways that alternative treatments can help all sorts of patients. That way, people who haven't tried methods beyond those of the Western medical establishment can begin to see the possibilities.

Normally, new patients are willing to try chiropractic only after the personal experience of a friend or family member. Until then, most had never even considered any other than the typical therapies. With that said, sometimes a book like this will find its way into someone's hands, and that person will be struck by his or her similarities to one of the patients described. When that happens, new worlds can open up for the reader.

What follows are a number of success stories. These are people who have come to me for help and whose experiences with chiropractic were so successful that when they heard I was writing a book, asked me to share their personal stories with all of you. Some of them filled out short forms to outline their situations in limited detail. Others preferred to share their complete stories, so we sat down together for longer interviews. This is merely a tiny example of the typical testimonials that you will find at any chiropractor's office!

I. Profiles

Success story #1: Sue

Major Complaint: I was suffering from severe neck and shoulder pain. The pain was negatively affecting my daily activities and personality. I also had very limited range of motion.

Past History: I have had neck pain and nerve damage in the past, resulting in cervical fusion four years prior to this incident. The surgery was successful in my estimation, but the pain never subsided 100%.

Other Doctors Consulted: M.D., Orthopedist, Neurologist, Physical Therapist. All doctors prescribed medications and additional surgery. The medications did not help and I am hesitant to have more surgery.

Chiropractic Results: Excellent! Dr. Paton reduced my pain from severe to manageable. My range of motion has dramatically improved. Additional attempts at further recovery and pain relief from acupuncture and bone stimulation had small results, leading me back for more chiropractic.

Success story #2: Ann

Major Complaint: Herniated T1-2, back disc. Severe back and leg pain.

Past History: Series of three epidural shots and physical therapy, oral medications, compromised lifestyle.

Other Doctors Consulted: M.D., Neurologist, Anesthesiologist, Physical Therapist. Doctors recommended I endure the pain until a spinal fusion was required. Surgery was the only option left.

Chiropractic Results: Then I met Dr. Paton! My life has changed completely. My pain level is minimal and I am on no medication. I am now "living" again. Dr. Paton truly is an angel on Earth. I am amazed at how such low-key and un-invasive treatment could be so effective.

Success story #3: Karen

Major Complaint: Back pain, sciatica
Past History: Back surgery, migraines, recent history of right shoulder pain.
Other Doctors Consulted: M.D., Orthopedist, Neurologist. Recommended more surgery (spinal fusion). I didn't want to do it.
Chiropractic Results: After seeking Dr. Paton's input, I am able to live pain-free for long periods of time. He is able to ease my acute flare-ups within days. I am using less pain medication. After having my back "fixed," Dr. Paton noticed my neck was out of line. He adjusted my neck and my migraines have decreased approximately 90%! Shoulder pain is non-existent when my neck is aligned.

Success story #4: Linda

Major Complaint: Fibromyalgia, strained muscles, lower back, mid-back and sciatic nerve pain. Severe headaches.
Past History: Fifteen different doctors. Limited movements affected my daily life.
Other Doctors Consulted: M.D., Orthopedist, Neurologist, Rheumatologist. Suggested physical therapy and water therapy.
Chiropractic Results: My life has become a lot easier to live. I have severe chronic pain. When it gets bad I call Dr. Paton, the miracle worker. My headaches go away immediately after adjustments.

Success story #5: Rusty

I had never met Scott Paton before I shuffled into his office in January 2005. My friend Kim had talked of a chiropractor she loved but I hadn't really paid much attention. But I had intractable, long-term back trouble, recently exacerbated by relocating our home from Connecticut to Florida. All those boxes! I had been to physical therapy most of the last summer. I was wearing a drugstore back brace. While all those things helped, the problem only retreated a little. It really did not go away.

Then one day I turned—maybe 15 degrees—and slightly coughed. The pain was spectacular. I went into muscle spasms. I could not sit down or stand. The pain was terrific. I called and asked if Dr. Paton had time. "Yes, of course. Come in." I would learn how real "*of course*" was later.

I could barely walk into Dr. Paton's office. I could not look up. I barely saw his face. But I heard his assurance. I felt his strong grip helping me into a chair and, ultimately, onto his treatment table. His adjustments began to help at once. A little at first. But they helped.

Dr. Paton never let go of the case, never stopped thinking of how to help me, always listened and, of course, adjusted. When I first got to Dr. Paton I could only walk with help—virtually I could not walk at all. Within days I was stepping on my own. Within a few weeks my walking *stride* was back.

Dr. Paton wants to reach out to patients to help them heal. He does just that in every way there is. I am very, very fortunate to have remembered the chiropractor my friend Kim had raved about. I'm truly blessed that I met Dr. Scott Paton.

Success story #6: Blanche

Dear Dr. Paton,

Our family would like to thank you for the care and friendship you extended to our mother, Blanche. Mom was your biggest cheerleader, always telling us what a wonderful doctor you were and how much better she felt after her treatments.

> *She always felt significantly better after a visit to
> your office. Her backaches and neck pains improved
> considerably due to your skills. Both her mental and
> emotional spirits were lifted. Thank you for the
> outstanding care and compassion shown to our Mom
> by you and your staff.*

Success story #7: Meghan

When Meghan was 3 months old, she was diagnosed with acid reflux and put on Zantac. Meghan still spit up a lot and was fussy and not sleeping well. At 5 months, I mentioned this to Dr. Paton and he adjusted her twice. Meghan is now sleeping well and has not spit up since her adjustment. She has been off Zantac for 3 months.

My 11-year-old daughter, Karianne, was diagnosed in February 2006 with growing pains. She was complaining that her foot hurt. X-rays showed no broken bones. Four weeks went by and it got worse. We ended up at the orthopedic doctor. He diagnosed her with Severs disease, which comes with growing pains. She wore heel cups in her shoes for months to supposedly fix the problem. By June she was still in pain and we went back to have an MRI done and found she had sprained part of her foot and stretched the ligaments. Her foot was put in a cast for 2 months.

Karianne was still in pain so we had Dr. Paton take a look. After 1½ months of adjusting her back, her hips (which we found were unevenly aligned by 3 or more inches), and her foot, Karianne was able to play sports again and participate in PE because she was no longer in pain.

During this time, I had been told by my primary doctor that I needed a spinal block and injections for my back. I decided to go to Dr. Paton instead. I was having pain from my TMJ also for the last 23 years and no one had been able to help.

When Dr. Paton told me he could help I was shocked and really did not believe him. After he adjusted my back I was pain-free and never needed the spinal block or injections and after adjusting my TMJ I was also pain-free! I was almost in tears thinking about how he'd been the only one to help me. Thank you, Dr. Paton, for helping my family get healthier and caring so much about us.

Success story #8: Gail

Major Complaint: Longstanding heel pain getting progressively worse, forcing me to ice 2-3 times daily; TMJ (dentist tried to alleviate with night guard). As the TMJ worsened, I've been wearing my night guard during the day also.

Chiropractic Results: On the first visit, Dr. Paton discovered a bone spur in my right heel. Within a week I was finished with daily icing. My jaw (TMJ) is also progressing very well. My night guard is reserved for sleeping. I never thought anything could be done for either condition. My treatments have made a tremendous improvement in my daily life.

Success story #9: Larry

Dear Dr. Paton,

As a new patient of yours within the last couple of weeks, and never having been to a chiropractor, I was more than a little apprehensive about the entire process and didn't quite know what to expect.

However, I knew I had to find an answer to what had become chronic neck, shoulder, and back pain following rotator cuff surgery in early 2004. I have always been very active, an avid runner and regular exerciser, so when I began having additional shooting pains that manifested themselves in the form of "shock" waves throughout my left torso, I knew I had to try something besides the usually prescribed mega-doses of anti-inflammatory drugs. The shock waves had intensified to the point that I was nearly brought to my knees when they struck. That is when I sought your help and advice.

After the initial visit, you were able to diagnose two areas of my spine that were obviously, from the x-rays, out of alignment. After a couple of follow-up adjustments, the shock waves subsided and have now been completely gone for over two weeks. In addition, the other chronic pains that I'd been learning to live with in my neck, shoulders, and back also began to subside. I have resumed my running routine, continued with the exercises you recommended, and have not felt this good in almost three years.

I'm still not sure exactly how you make this entire process of alignments and adjustments work, but I am now a believer. Thanks again for all that you do.

Success story #10: Gerrit

I was experiencing severe pain in my right ankle that was making physical activity almost impossible. My first reaction was to see a podiatrist. They took x-rays of my ankle and foot and could not make a diagnosis of what the problem was. The podiatrist insisted that my only alternative would be aggressive treatment, starting with an expensive MRI and possibly surgery.

Aggressive treatment was not what I wanted to do. I decided to give chiropractic medicine a try with Dr. Paton. As a professional basketball player, I wanted someone who was familiar with sports medicine and Dr. Paton has experience with many other sports programs in the area.

On my first visit, Dr. Paton sat me down and we came up with a plan to correct my ankle injury by aligning my neck, back, as well as ankle. Within the second week I noticed a substantial difference, and after the third week the pain in my ankle was gone. I have been extremely happy with what Dr. Paton has done for me and would highly recommend chiropractic as a smart alternative to other expensive and aggressive treatments.

Success story #11: Seth

Major Complaint: Fell while wakeboarding on the lake. Initial impact was to the right side of my face. **Problems:** Dizziness; shortness of breath; rapid heart rate; blurred vision; numbness in hands and

arms; muscle cramps; hearing and 25-lb. weight loss.
Other Doctors Consulted: I saw my primary care physician six times, had three different sets of blood work. On the first visit it was found that I had broken right eardrum and that was the cause of the dizziness. During two months I was in the ER three different times for dizziness, shortness of breath, numbness and rapid heartbeat. I had blood work done twice, received an IV for dehydration, CT scan of the head, and was put on a heart monitor for 24 hours. The results were all normal, including that the eardrum had healed within the first week of the accident

I saw an ENT physician three weeks after the accident; results were normal. I saw an optometrist within the first month with normal results. I also saw a dentist after eight weeks; revealed two fractured teeth on the right.

Chiropractic Results: On the first visit after x-rays were done, Dr. Paton discovered there was a problem with my C1-2 vertebrae. After two weeks of seeing Dr. Paton, I was able to return to work and the majority of my symptoms were diminishing. I have been under his care for two months and am making great progress with every visit.

II. Interviews

Interview #1: Devlin 9 *(4-year-old boy with Cerebral Palsy)*

DR. PATON: [to Devlin's mother, Edie] *Can you tell us a little bit about Devlin?*

EDIE: Devlin was a 26-week preemie. He weighed 1 lb., 1 oz. at birth and had a gram-negative infection that killed his older brother and almost killed him. [Note: Gram-negative meningitis, more common in infants than adults, is an infection of the membranes covering the brain and spinal cord (meninges) caused by gram-negative bacteria (bacteria that turn pink when exposed to a special stain).] He's almost four years old now.

When we started seeing Dr. Paton, Devlin had "chicken-wing arms" and frozen joints. We've had excellent results bringing Devlin to Dr. Paton, in all Devlin's extremities. Dr. Paton keeps all his joints moving. His rehab doctor is very happy with the way things are going, too. By now, had we not come to Paton, all Devlin's joints would be frozen. But now his chicken-wing arms straighten out.

And every time Devlin comes in he gives Dr. Paton a big smile; he's so happy to be here. Normally he's screams and hollers at other doctors' offices. He has nothing to do with any other doctor. He's always smiling and laughing when he comes out from seeing you, Dr. Paton. I can't say enough about you and your treatment here.

DR. PATON: *You got some resistance about sending Devlin here, didn't you?*

EDIE: Yes, I had a physical therapist who told me that if I brought Devlin to a chiropractor that she would quit treating him because if anything happened she wouldn't know if it were her fault or the chiropractor's fault. So I chose to come to you. And it's been so helpful, it's been worth it.

DR. PATON: *Thank you, I'm honored. I think you told me you were expecting resistance from the rehab doctor, too, but he supported your decision to come here, is that right?*

EDIE: Yes, he was very happy. When he saw how well Devlin was doing and I told him he was coming here, he said, "Keep doing it, then."

DR. PATON: *That's fabulous. It's nice to know that there are open minds. So many people think chiropractors treat only neck and low back pain. Besides the joints moving better, do you notice any other effects from chiropractic?*

EDIE: Devlin arches a lot less and his arms are moving all the time now. When I first started coming here, they weren't moving at all. I was a little surprised at how gentle the manipulations were, too. Devlin didn't smile much before coming here. It's wonderful to see Devlin smile so much now.

Interview #2: Jan

Jan has been a patient of mine for three years. She initially presented with back pain. When she came to me for help, she'd spent three months on her back and was concerned about getting better. I started treating her but also referred her to an integrative/holistic medical doctor for her all-around care.

DR. PATON: *What is it about chiropractic that you like the most?*

JAN: My philosophy is that I have always chosen to have preventative healthcare rather than "treatment." But last year I became very sick and spent three months on my back. I knew I had to make the decision between typical medical intervention and alternative care. And now, between my holistic integrative care and chiropractic care, I'm totally up and around. You only have to look at my x-rays to see the difference between what I looked like then compared to how I am now.

My son has also come to you for treatment for allergies. Every time he comes to see, you it's like night and day when you compare how he looks and feels when he goes into the office and then how he looks and feels when he leaves. Within 24 hours there's not one symptom of an allergy. I know now that that makes sense because every single point on the body is linked to the spine.

DR. PATON: *How do you respond to people's reactions when you tell them you use chiropractic—for yourself and your children?*

JAN: Actually, a man I referred to you this past week made the comment that chiropractors are quacks. And I said, "But you're sitting there in excruciating pain and you haven't been to see one. And your wife was in pain; she just went to see one and she's not in pain anymore. Your daughter went to see one and *she's* not in pain anymore. It seems to me that you might benefit yourself." My attitude is: Give it a try, what have you got to lose? And that's what I try to convey to people.

I have to say, though, that you are the first chiropractor who has taken the time to show me what you're doing and why. You've taken the x-rays and said, "Here's where we are now; this is what we're going to do to correct these things," instead of telling me, "This is what you've got…we'll just try to maintain it." In the course of having a previous chiropractor for three years and now you for three years, my x-rays show that you have corrected the problem. You can see it on the x-rays and I can feel it in how well I feel.

Interview #3: Kirstin (age 12)
Kirstin came in complaining of headaches and a new diagnosis of ADHD.

DR. PATON: *What kind of treatment had you had for your headaches prior to seeing me?*

KRISTIN: Nothing, really.

DR. PATON: *Were you taking any medications?*

KRISTIN: No.

DR. PATON: *How often were you getting headaches and how long did you have them?*

KRISTIN: I had them every day for a couple of months. It was hard to study and focus or read.

DR. PATON: *Did you tell the pediatrician?*

KRISTIN'S MOM: The doctors were talking about giving her medication for the ADD and sending her to a neurologist and then one of her teachers mentioned that she sees a chiropractor. I was already a patient here so I brought Kirstin to see you.

DR. PATON: *So you heard from Kirstin's teacher that ADD could be helped by chiropractic?*

MOM: Yes.

DR. PATON: *Does it hurt to get adjusted, Kirstin?*

KRISTIN: No. I like it.

DR. PATON: *Would you recommend other kids see a chiropractor?*

KRISTIN: Yeah.

DR. PATON: *Have you had many headaches lately?*

KRISTIN: No. They totally went away without any medication.

DR. PATON: *Did your grades go up?*

KRISTIN: Actually, yeah. And now I just come once a month.

Interview #4: Larry *(age 40)*

Larry presented with multiple problems, including severe weight loss, neck and back pain, and inability to sleep due to pain. Before giving you Larry's own version of what happened when he came to see me, I'd like to add a brief introduction.

Larry is a wonderful, happy person, but you would never have known it. You see, initially, he wasn't very pleasant to be around. Truth be told, he was miserable and let everyone around him know it.

I first heard about Larry from his Mom, Evelyn. Evelyn was referred to my office by another patient and was looking for help with her knee. She had hit dead end after dead end, and no other healthcare facility seemed to be able to help her. She was told that she had arthritis, and to "live with it or get a knee replacement."

At her initial exam I took x-rays and then explained that we'd be adjusting her lower back to correct for misalignments, which would ultimately help her knee. I showed her how misalignments of her back were inextricably related to the problems she was having in her knee, how it was all "connected." I further explained that we'd be adjusting her knee as needed to speed the healing process.

Evelyn was skeptical at first, but agreed to proceed with care. I stressed that this would not be an overnight fix and that correcting misalignments took time. I set her up for approximately twenty to twenty-five visits and urged her to make every appointment. Evelyn stated that making appointments might be tough, as her schedule was difficult.

Early in her care, Evelyn stated that she wasn't seeing the results that she expected. I repeated what I'd said on her first visit, that based on her exam and x-rays she'd need approximately twenty to twenty-five treatments to stabilize her condition and achieve the results we were after. I couldn't help adding, trying to be patient, that if I'd expected she'd be better in only six visits, I would have told her six visits! She cautiously agreed to continue her care but I could see that she was doubting herself, me, and the process.

Then, a miracle! At around the twelfth visit, her knee pain was starting to recede! By the eighteenth visit, it was gone altogether! At this point, I had not only gained her trust, but her respect. She began telling all of her friends about our office and about chiropractic. And that's when she told me about her son, Larry.

Evelyn spoke solemnly and sincerely. In fact, she started to tear up as she talked. "You have to help my son Larry," she said, "because if you don't, he's going to die." My first thought was perhaps she was being a bit melodramatic about her son's health dilemma. But I soon realized that wasn't the case at all.

She told me about how Larry was taking all kinds of medication and was losing weight in dangerous proportions. Normally a fit 145 pounds, Larry's weight was now down to below 120. She told me that he was having such a tough time, he was forced to come to live with his mother for help and support.

Evelyn begged me not to say anything to Larry about treatment if he ever came to the office with her, that he didn't believe in chiropractic and would storm out (if she was lucky enough to even get him to come with her in the first place). She told me that the only thing he was getting from his doctors at this point was more and more drugs, and she was sure I was the only person who would be able to save his life. At that point, Evelyn vowed to get him in to see me and that she would do whatever it took.

Within a few days, Evelyn had another appointment with me and reiterated the fact that she emphatically did not want me to say a word about anything she'd said. I assured her that everything was in the strictest confidence.

Time after time, she urged Larry to come to the office with her, at least for a consultation. But she was right: Larry flatly refused to even come to the office. He didn't think that any doctor would be able to help him and that chiropractors were "quacks" (I later found this out from Larry). Then one day, another miracle occurred. Evelyn needed to get her car repaired and Larry was driving her around. On this particularly day, Evelyn coincidentally had an appointment at my office and, after the visit, planned to go a few doors down to pick up her dry cleaning. Unfortunately, her dry cleaning wouldn't be ready for another hour. Enter Larry.

I was taken aback when I first saw this man. He looked thin and sickly and his skin had a uniquely disturbing hue. Its color was literally gray, like an ashtray.

Somehow between Evelyn and me, we managed to convince Larry to have me take a look at him. I took him through the standard questionnaire, then an exam and x-rays. He was very abrupt with his answers and I could tell he had no interest in being at my office. Our office prides itself on being very upbeat and we didn't let Larry's attitude rub us the wrong way. I was just pleased that Larry was actually having a consult at all, and continued trying to get the information I needed to provide care—*if* he'd let me.

Larry did ultimately return to me for help, but instead of my telling you the story, I'm going to let him tell it himself from his own point of view:

DR. PATON: Can you tell us a bit about yourself, Larry?

L: My background is that I've been living in Los Angeles. First I raised private capital for movies. I found I liked working around the actual film production more than raising money, so I starting to do producing and directing. I tried acting, too, but didn't really like that much. I wanted to find movies and make them happen. I became the VP of a movie company called Living Element. I started to work with animators, directors, producers…and I knew this was what I wanted to do.

The problem was that even though I did very well and they paid me a lot of cash, there were a lot of internal problems in the work and I ended up going from one company to the next looking for the right position. I still made a lot of money but it was a very stressful time.

About a year and a half ago, a friend of mine said, "You've got to stop right now and start doing what you want to do. You're making lots of money but you're never happy." And he was right. Plus, by that point, I was taking amazing amounts of drugs that my doctor was prescribing.

I have to be honest with you, too. I was smoking weed all the time. I was taking everything I could think of to make myself feel better, but it didn't matter what it was, nothing helped. I even tried cocaine, desperately trying to feel better, mentally and physically. I had two problems: my frame of mind and my physical well-being, both a result of the life I was living.

The truth is, I hated the life I was living. I was in constant pain—physical pain; my neck hurt constantly, and my back, and I had headaches all the time…and all that pain made me very, very angry all the time. I used to relate it to Chinese water torture, because what drives you insane is that it never stops. I could never feel good or relax. I drank heavily—anything for relief. And drinking helped. I drank and was out of pain for a while so I'd drink more. I think that's why a lot of people drink too much.

I couldn't change my frame of mind and couldn't change the way I felt physically. But I was successful. And that's what was so confusing. But finally one day I sat down on the couch and told my wife, "I'm making $50,000 a month and I've never been unhappier in my life. I'm in constant pain and nothing solves it. I can't do this anymore." At first she said, "You can't walk away from a job making that kind of money." But I said, "I'm going to. I'm not living my life like this anymore. I want to be happy. I don't want to be the richest guy in the world. I want to be the happiest guy in the world."

My wife wasn't happy about my changing my life and I knew it was about the money. I felt she didn't care about me or my well-being. Eventually we agreed to divorce. I was driving her back to the East Coast when things really changed for me. On the way, my friend David (the one who got me to admit how miserable I was) spoke to me about what I was doing. He told me he thought I should either be producing music or movies. I said, "If you give me the money to start a company, I'll do that and I'll run the company."

We sat down and talked about what made us happy and both of us agreed that we really liked Garth Brooks. We both knew that Brooks was someone who loved what he did. David reminded me that success isn't just measured by wealth; it's measured by how you feel. He told me he thought a lot of my physical problems derived from mental problems.

I told him I was going to change my life that day, that I was going to walk away from the job I had. And I did. I went back to L.A. and, with David's help, started my own company, doing my own stuff.

At that point, my mental pain left—I was really feeling happier—but I still had the physical pain, which was getting worse and worse. And that bummed me out…here I'm doing what I want to do and I'm still unhappy because I'm still in pain all the time. Half the problem was better but the other half was overwhelming me. I was sleeping only two hours at a time, no matter what I did.

So I decided to terminate my whole L.A. experience for a couple of months, go to an entirely different place, see my mother…maybe if I got out of there something magical would happen. I was getting violently sick all the time and I knew I had to do something. I wanted to see my mother because I really thought I'd be dead in a month.

My mother started to tell me about you as soon as I got there. The last time I saw her she couldn't walk, in November. Then when I came back to see her in February of this year, she was walking fine. I asked her how it happened and she said, "This chiropractor has changed my whole life." I couldn't believe it. "You went to a chiropractor?" "Yes," she said, "and you need to go, too." I said, "He can't help me, nobody can help me." After all, I'd been to doctors and taken every drug there is. I didn't want to do any of it anymore. I argued with her and refused to go.

One day my mother's car happened to be in a shop to be fixed and she needed a ride to go to see you. While we were there, she kept saying, "Since we're here…since you're already here…why don't you just go talk to Dr. Paton and see what he'll say?" I knew if I didn't I'd never hear the end of it; my mother would harp on it forever. So I said I'd see you one time just to prove she was wrong. I said, "This guy's a quack, give me a break. He's not going to help me. If my *medical* doctor can't help me, how can this guy? He doesn't even have a medical license."

So I filled out the forms, listened to you, and didn't believe a word you told me. I left, went back to my Mom's, and told her I wasn't going to go back. She told me I'd promised her that I'd try. I told her that if she'd start taking vitamins, doing some of the things I wanted her to do, that I would go a couple more times. But I said, "I'm only going to do it to show you it's a bunch of you-know-what, a waste of time. Will that make you happy?" She said yes. So I started to see you, but I had no hope at all that you would do anything except take my money.

I had told someone while I was still in L.A. that I'd rather kill myself than live like that with constant pain. When you've been in so much pain for so long, you just want it to end…you can't stand it anymore. There's such a thing as living and there's existing. I didn't want to exist—I wanted to live.

DR. PATON: You said you saw a primary care doctor, a former cardiologist, right?

LARRY: Yes, he said he chose not to practice cardiology anymore because lawsuits were too common so he just went into general practice.

DR. PATON: *Originally you saw him because of your neck and back pain?*

LARRY: Yeah. But he told me that the way my body was configured was the way I was born and that there was nothing he could do for me. He said unless I wanted surgery, the only thing he could suggest was medication. He told me to just take the drugs and deal with the pain.

DR. PATON: *But then he put you on thyroid medicine based on a blood test. What was that for?*

LARRY: He said it was a good idea to do a blood test to see what else might be wrong. So he did a routine blood test, which showed an abnormal thyroid. For that he gave me Synthroid and that's when I started feeling really anxious, so they tried to offset that with more drugs. I was taking Vicadins, muscle relaxers and Xanax, a tranquilizer.

DR. PATON: *I'm dumbfounded.*

LARRY: I had so much anxiety and the drugs did work but they zombified me. My son always knew I was on tranquilizers when he talked to me. He said, "You're not you. I'm not talking to *you*. You're nothing like who you are when you're taking those drugs. You should stop taking them."

I said, "But my doctor's prescribing them. He's a doctor, he should know." What was I supposed to do? Who was I supposed to go to? Doctors are supposed to help you. He was prescribing the drugs and I did feel more relaxed. My son said, "Yeah, but you're not coherent, you're only half there." But I just assumed that was the price I had to pay to lose the pain and anxiety I had.

The back pain was still pretty severe, though, so I told the doctor the Vicadins didn't work anymore. He told me I was probably becoming addicted to Vicadin so he'd give me morphine. When my son found out about that, he told me not to take them. My answer: "My doctor told me to take them, so I'm going to." And I did.

DR. PATON: *Didn't you get some shots for your back pain, too?*

LARRY: Yeah, from the same doctor. He used a big needle and put it in my back and twisted it around. I can't remember what it was. I was so wasted on stuff I have no idea what he was giving me. Then the last thing he gave me was morphine tablets.

DR. PATON: *Morphine?*

LARRY: They didn't help, though. They didn't really do that much. I had to go to five pharmacies just to find one that carried it because it's hard to get. I didn't realize you're supposed to have all kinds of tests to take it—you've got to be seriously ill to take it. I just took what he told me to take. And that's when I started to question what I was doing. I started reading about morphine and talking to my son about it. He's the one who told me how serious the drug was...

And I knew that this doctor was just a drug dealer with a medical license. I would walk up to his office and say, "I need some Vicadins and muscle relaxers." "You need to see the doctor?" "No." "Okay." And they'd just hand me prescriptions and I'd walk away. I can call right now and tell him what I want and he'd say okay. He wouldn't ask me why or to come and see him. My son would tell me it was impossible, but it was totally possible. I could get anything, try anything. He'd just write the prescription.

And he'd send false statements to my insurance company. He'd bill them for all kinds of things he never did. Nails in my foot, wheezing...and all he was doing was giving me prescription drugs. Anything I wanted. "I'll take 50 of those, 100 of those and 75 of those." He'd give me so many drugs my friends would want to buy them from me. I didn't want to sell my friends the drugs, but I told them to go see this "doctor" and they would, and they'd get whatever they wanted.

But the drugs were only killing my desire and drive. I forced myself to go to work but it was killing my ambition. I knew I wasn't all I could be but I was under a fog I couldn't get out from under. There was never a solution, just more drugs.

DR. PATON: *And that's when you came to see your Mom?*

LARRY: That's right. I said to myself, "The next thing this guy will tell me is to take heavier morphine and then I'll be addicted to morphine and I know where that's going." I had to be honest. I could feel it was killing me to take the drugs. I could feel my body was telling me to stop taking them, that I was dying. I didn't want to eat anymore. I didn't care. That's when my weight started dropping. I had given up on life.

I actually saw a show on the Discovery Channel where a kid, nineteen, lost so much weight he actually died. Only nineteen. And I said, "That's exactly what I'm doing. I'm withering away. I'm going to die if I don't change." I prayed my mother would help me. I knew there was something that would happen, I didn't know what it was, but I hoped it would happen when I got here.

DR. PATON: *You know, your Mom told me before you came in, "My son's going to die. Please don't tell him I told you this, because he'll get mad at me, but you need to see him and he needs to see you."*

LARRY: After it was all over, she said, "I knew you were dying and I didn't know what to do about it." She kept saying, when I was still in L.A., "Come and see me, come and see me." And my son said the same thing. I knew I had to reverse the process, but I didn't know how. I'd tried every drug there is. I had no confidence in doctors anymore. I was convinced no one could help me. But I was wrong.

DR. PATON: When did you start to feel better?

LARRY: It was a slow process. But slowly, slowly, I started slowly feeling better. I could tell. There was a day when I knew things were starting to change. I just had that feeling. You told me it would take a while, but I thought you told me that so you could bleed me of as much cash as you could get, not because that's what it takes.

But I couldn't deny that something was changing, and it wasn't only physical, it was emotional. Of course I told myself I was just having a good day so I wouldn't give you any credit.

Then another week went by and I felt better and I felt better on a more regular basis. Then I started feeling better just walking around in general. Then one day I went to bed and I woke up the next day and it was 9 a.m. I'd slept through the entire night. I was amazed—but convinced myself that could have been a fluke, too. But it happened over and over. Then one night I was lying in bed and realized my neck didn't hurt. I thought, *When I lie here it doesn't bother me. And my back isn't hurting anymore either. I'm not in pain like I was before.*

One day I just noticed it. These things usually hurt and irritate me and they weren't bothering me anymore. I could feel myself getting stronger. And then my desire to be healthier came back because I wasn't in pain.

Then my mother said to me, "You don't have the anger you had a month or two ago." I said, "I'm not in pain all the time. I don't have any reason to be angry anymore. I don't have anything against the world to be angry about. I can think more clearly, too." And I know it might be strange to say but I actually feel I'm getting smarter, too.

My whole being is changing in a good way; I'm getting stronger and stronger. When I used to work out I had shoulder pain all the time—I did it anyway and worked through the pain—but now there's no pain whatsoever in my neck or my back or shoulders...even when I do weights. The more I came and saw you, the better I felt. Just like you told me I would but I didn't believe you.

And I know now I'm going to be healthier and stronger than I've ever felt in my life. I can feel my body doing something...something's happening. And I'm not taking drugs. My anxiety level has dropped dramatically. I don't scream and holler for no reason. I'm off the drug that you told me was causing that and all those things are gone. This is the most amazing thing I've ever had done in my life. I cannot believe that I'm not taking drugs or getting injections, I'm not taking prescription drugs, and the problems are all going away—all of them.

I told my mother at the beginning, "I'll bet you I'll wake up tomorrow and be back where I was," and I felt that way for a week or two, thinking it would all end. I thought, *You mean I can feel great?* I've never felt great for more than a day or two my entire adult life. The pain and suffering always returned. But it hasn't yet and she told me it would get better and better and better.

DR. PATON: *Everyone has exacerbations or flare-ups—I guess you'd have to call it life—but now I see you only once every month or every few months, right? Once your spine is in alignment and nerves are working again, it takes a quick adjustment and you're right back to where you were.*

LARRY: Yeah, it just takes a quick adjustment and I'm back to where I was. And the coolest part of all is living a life without pain.

CHAPTER SEVENTEEN

FAITH

What faith means to me

For many people, faith is an important part of the healing process—not just religious faith but a belief in the ways of the universe and in signs that things will get better.

Remember the story about when I was working in the men's department of Dillard's after college and felt uncomfortable about not exhibiting what I believed to be the manifestations of "success"? I have thought about that time often through the years, and have since come to learn that it is our focus on the obstacles we encounter that actually seems to will them to occur, or prevents us from moving in the right direction altogether.

After not having gotten the job I wanted as a medical rep, I eventually got a position with Westinghouse Remediation Services (WRS), an environmental subsidiary to the large corporation, Westinghouse. It was a career that allowed me to use my chemistry degree—a better fit than the other job. If you remember, they were also the ones who were paying for my Master's program. Had you asked me a few months earlier if I could see a better future, I would have categorically told you NO. But just a short while later, I was doing pretty well.

The job kept me traveling all over the state and although occasionally I took a flight, the majority was done by car. I had suffered from dull low back pain for years and kept the flare-ups under control with Advil as needed, but all the driving really started to exacerbate my low back pain. Then, an interesting thing happened—a sort of proverbial "crossroads of life" moment.

I was at a routine yearly physical exam that was mandatory for my job. The doctor gave me a clean bill of health then asked if I had any other concerns. I let him know about my dull back pain, then he looked at me, leaned down and whispered, "I'm not supposed to be doing this, the clinic director wouldn't approve of it, but lie down on your side and I'll manipulate your low back. It'll make it feel better."

I did as he instructed. The doctor pushed on my back, and poof! I felt great. I was amazed! Why hadn't I known about this sooner? I had mentioned my pain to other doctors in the past, but had only been given medication and more medication. This doctor told me that he was a D.O., a doctor of osteopathy. He added that chiropractors do this kind of thing all the time and they call it an adjustment.

I was excited about my new discovery. I had known nothing at all at that time about chiropractors or their methods, but now I had made a connection between sore backs and chiropractic adjustments. It was like getting a huge universal tap on the shoulder. Suddenly it was all I could think about and I knew at the most fundamental level that I had found my calling. Now, I couldn't be more grateful for that cosmic shove!

Another piece of the story

I struggled over the decision of whether to include "faith" as a topic in a book about health and medicine, anticipating that some subjects may put off potential readers. I asked myself over and over, "Don't I want to reach as many people as possible? What if some people might not read this book because I mention my faith and my beliefs?"

The answer to these questions took a while in coming. In fact, it was only when I recently took my family on a trip to Caladesi Island, a little island off the coast of Clearwater, Florida, that I got my answer loud and clear.

Having had five appearances in the list of "top ten beaches in the country," Caladesi made it all the way to number two—twice. Caladesi Island is a very special place, one where you can really relax. We drove our boat right up to the island and planned to spend the night because it closes at dusk to visitors. We plugged into shore power and my wife, three children and I set about to have a peaceful night.

As I lay in the bed of the boat, my wife and kids sound asleep, listening to the sounds of the island and feeling the cool breeze the boat rock with the gentle waves, I was surprised to find I couldn't sleep. I couldn't stop thinking about the skeptics, the people I wouldn't be able to reach, the ones who wouldn't want to be reached. I thought about the people who would laugh at my vision of health-care and my mention of "faith," or denounce what I had to say.

I wondered about what I should leave in or out of the book to assuage certain factions. Would I alienate more people than I would reach by my honesty and expressing all I think and feel relative to our current healthcare system, chiropractic and alternative methods of treatment?

With all these thoughts swirling around in my head, I knew there was only one thing I could. And that was to look to my faith and trust that the answers would come.

To give you some background, I will share with you that I am a devout and dedicated Christian who tries to live that lifestyle to the best of my ability. I have a profound and deep belief in God (and in Jesus as His only son). But over the years I have opened my mind (and heart) to philosophies I previously knew nothing about as I progressed through the maze of trying to treat patients as best I could. I looked at all the options, asked questions and began to realize that one's religion does not necessarily exclude integrating tools and techniques from other cultures, nor does doing so mean giving up one's own cultural, religious or ethical beliefs.

So as I tossed and turned that night on the boat, I asked for guidance to know that I would be doing the right thing in sharing the whole picture—*my* whole picture. I prayed and finally I fell asleep, the most peaceful sleep I've ever had, with the waves splashing against the boat.

The next day we were up early. My children were as excited as could be, looking for shells, and I found myself smiling, enjoying my kids' excitement in the simple pleasures that life has to offer.

At that time of morning, the beach was virtually deserted—quiet and serene. As I walked, I heard the words, "This is the path to global peace, love and happiness," and I knew they were referring to my efforts to bring people together in a loving, peaceful way through the integrated forms of both Eastern and Western medicine and philosophies.

I thought about how I had started down a path previously unknown to me, how I had studied chiropractic instead of pursuing another career. I thought about all the messages I was getting in my daily life through work in the field of healing. I knew that I would keep getting those messages—and that this was one of them.

As I walked, I asked silently, "How do I know it's you, God? How do I know it's the right thing to do?" And the voice said, "Look around, that's the answer." And I did. I looked at the most beautiful beach on this most beautiful day. I felt the breeze, saw the swaying palm trees, heard the sounds of the waves and the wildlife…

And I knew that it was the right thing to do.

The link

Now I want to share another story to show how the Universe nudges us toward unknown things—and that, if we keep an open heart and mind, our receptiveness will be rewarded. In this case, it's a story about how I came to learn of the de-stressing techniques practiced in other cultures, and how I've incorporated these into my daily life to achieve a more peaceful, balanced state.

It's too bad I had no knowledge of these techniques prior to a trip my wife and I made to Greece, where I would be speaking at the 2004 pre-Olympic Scientific Congress. I was always uncomfortable with public speaking and this group would be larger than ever before. In addition, the audience was made up of professionals whom I very much wanted to impress.

During our non-direct flight, somewhere between JFK Airport and Greece, one of my suitcases was lost—the one with all my clothes for the presentation, plus some of my handwritten notes for my speech. My anxiety level skyrocketed. I felt as if I might have a literal heart attack. My wife tried her best to calm me down but I was having none of it. The way my brain was hard-wired back then, I resented and felt patronized by any words of encouragement from anyone who had not been in my shoes. I felt like saying to her, "How can you say everything's going to be okay?! You don't know what I'm going through!"

I know my outlook was that of a victim: "Why me? Why on this occasion? Why not someone else or some other day?" It was only after Janice (the saint of patience) called the airline and they assured me the bag would be delivered late that evening that I finally calmed down a bit. Janice persuaded me to leave the hotel for dinner at a beautiful restaurant on the water, where we ate traditional Greek food and gazed out at the beautiful vista.

The hour we spent at the restaurant was a nice stress relief but truth be told, it was short-lived and I couldn't really appreciate the beauty of the landscape or the joy of being with my wife. I was in too big a hurry to get back to the hotel, where I proceeded to drink cup after cup of strong coffee to stay awake while I waited in the lobby for my suitcase. I needed that bag in my hands in order to feel better, and nothing could persuade me otherwise.

The upshot, of course, was that the suitcase did eventually arrive, complete with my notes and clothes. But since then I've asked myself many times how things might have been different had I reacted differently—perhaps with annoyance tempered by a sense of humor and the knowledge that somehow things would be right in the end. I know it would have been better for me physically and emotionally. The stress had taken a toll on me *and* my wife.

The next morning, Janice and I went to see the hall where I would be speaking. Unaware that it was occupied, we walked in to find an auditorium full of people intently listening to a presentation and periodically performing some type of deep breathing exercise that involved raising their arms as they inhaled then quickly lowering them as they forcefully exhaled. The exercises were being led by a gentleman with a calm voice, speaking in English with a German accent. Janice wanted to leave because she felt we were being rude by walking into a lecture after it had started, but I suggested we stay.

It turned out that the lecturer represented a group called The Art of Living Foundation, and my exposure to its teachings hours before my lecture would have a startling effect on my ability to present that day...in fact, it would literally change my life.

The Art of Living teaches techniques in meditation to help people in their efforts to battle daily stress and achieve well-being. Not having been exposed to any form of meditation before, Janice and I looked at each other skeptically. But since we were coincidentally so stressed out that day, we decided to give it a chance. What did we have to lose?

We both listened and took part in the exercises. Afterwards, the woman next to us began to chat with us, and the lecturer came over to introduce himself. Christof had an incredible way about him—he exuded kindness and friendliness. Janice and I both felt very relaxed while talking to him. We had a short, get-to-know-each-other conversation and he invited Janice, me, and Ritsa, the woman next to us, to a free expanded meditation session.

We all agreed to meet the next day after my speech. Christof was excited to hear that I would be lecturing and asked if he could attend. I said I'd be glad to see him there and told him that I was excited but nervous about the presentation.

Before we left, Ritsa, who was from Crete, invited us on a private tour of the local monasteries. We began at a large monastery and were disappointed to find it locked. We decided to walk around anyway to get a feel for the place when, suddenly, a very old woman came around the corner. She spoke to Ritsa in Greek and Ritsa whispered that this was the caretaker of the church.

The caretaker opened the door to the church and allowed us to enter. Inside, we smelled the stalest, oldest, mustiest smell that I've ever experienced, and I could tell Janice agreed by the way she was wrinkling her nose. There were no lights, only candles, and it was very dark except for the slivers of sunlight entering through the windows.

The short, hunchbacked caretaker pointed to an old wooden podium and told Ritsa that a portion of the Bible, Thessalonians in the New Testament, had been written there. It wasn't clear if the podium had always been in that particular church or had been transferred there but either way, we felt an energetic connection to the spirit in that place and were moved by it.

The following day, after a somewhat difficult night of alternately sleeping fitfully and lying awake, thinking about my presentation, I walked into the conference room. It was packed! I started to sweat. Janice wished me luck and I went up to the stage, hoping I didn't look as nervous as I felt.

Up there, I could see the names and countries written on the tags of people sitting in the front row, and I found myself focusing on this as if it were the most critical information I'd ever seen: China, Denmark, Japan, Australia. Some of the audience members had digital or video cameras and I stood before them, shaking like a leaf. Then I saw Christof in the back of the audience. His face was calm, smiling, unperturbed, and it helped me relax enough to take a deep breath. Though I didn't know the first thing about the concept of vibratory alignment then, I know now that's what was going on when I locked onto Christof's face. Somehow, then, I pulled myself together and began my talk.

Afterwards, incredibly relieved, I got ready for our meditation session. As Christians, Janice and I were somewhat guarded as we approached the class. We'd heard all the stories about "New Age-y" and subculture cults. We were suspicious, having never questioned the premise on which these cultures were based, and had grouped all types of "meditation" in with lots of other philosophies. Because we liked Christof, however, and I felt he'd had a positive effect on my ability to focus and present, we decided to go in. When we entered, Christof immediately congratulated me on my speech then introduced us to the group. Janice and I were the only two Americans.

Class began with the same breathing techniques Christof had been doing the day before. After a few minutes, these were expanded to very relaxing deep-breathing exercises. Still, I was filled with apprehension. What if this involved some type of religion that prayed to a god other than my God? What if they would try to exert some kind of influence on us—hypnotize us, or extract money from us? My mind was racing.

Soon, my thoughts were off and running: I should have practiced more before my lecture…if only I'd listened to Janice when she suggested certain changes. Why did I treat her the way I did just because I was so frustrated? In fact, why did I treat people badly sometimes? What did *I* do to deserve to be treated like that when I was a teenager…and on and on.

Not yet satisfied with the misery I had created in myself, I began to worry about the future as well as the past. Will I be able to afford to send my kids to college? What will I do if I can't lose the weight I want? Believe me, if you saw my external self, sitting quietly, breathing in concert with the people around me, you would have been shocked to hear the scenarios of doubt that were parading through my head. I felt powerless to stop them, though I wanted to.

Finally, I don't know how much time went by but I started to lose the thread of my negative thinking. I heard myself breathing instead. As I listened to the air flowing in and out, I felt myself grow calmer. I realized that thinking these thoughts had not accomplished one single thing—other than keeping me locked in a state of panic and negativity.

After all, I had not solved any problems or faced any challenges; certainly I had not found the money to send my children to college or lost the weight. I felt a little shaken. Did this mean that worrying over these issues was irrelevant? If that were the case, I would need to rethink a lot of the ways I thought in general. And that was a really big idea to consider.

This experience was the start of how Janice and I changed our thinking and the way we lived our lives. What we learned is that we have constant issues that enter our mind; they swing back and forth like a pendulum: one swing over to all the things we regret from our past and then one swing in the other direction, to all the things we worry about in the future. Unfortunately, the more negative these thoughts are, the harder they are to ignore…in fact, the more they tend to hang around. We dwell on the past and let anxiety guide us—or misguide us—into the future. Stress ensues and continues to build and build and build.

We have developed our own way of thinking about this destructive tendency, which helps us visualize the process and turn it around. We see and hear our thoughts and consciously visualize this pendulum, swinging back and forth. Then we gradually slow the pendulum down to a complete stop. The time and place where it comes to a full rest represents the true present—and in the present, there is no regret about the past and no worry about the future. Some call it living in "the now," an expression I had discarded as a foolish platitude until I actually started experiencing it! Our goal in meditation is to get into that present, where we temporarily forget about the past and leave the future to unfold without anxiety.

Of course, living life means you can't forget about the past and ignore the future. But that's exactly why taking a few moments a day to live in the present, to stop the swing of the pendulum, alleviates stress to the degree that you can deal with whatever life dishes out.

This is accomplished through deep breathing or meditation as well as through physical exercise. Both are ways to push the pause button on your life, to relax. In the process, you stop consciously *thinking*. There is no need to pray; there is no "need" at all. For this short period of time, you are in a completely relaxed state of mind, which refuels you for what's coming next. My own "meditations" generally last about thirty minutes and I wake feeling truly refreshed.

In the end, Christof and the Art of Living were simply promoting a way to feel peace and relaxation through meditation. That's it: no deity worship, no cult, no monetary solicitations. And Janice and I both have to admit feeling a renewed sense of connectedness—to each other, our family and our lives.

It sure would have been nice to have met Christof before the airlines lost my luggage that day, but the experience nonetheless led me toward living a life of happiness. Now I recommend taking an Art of Living course to many of my patients (www.artofliving.org) in order to help them open their minds to find new ways to feel productive and healthy.

> *"Spiritual blossoming means expanding in all dimensions—being happy, at ease with yourself and everybody around you"*
> —Sri Sri Ravi Shankar, Founder of the Art of Living Foundation

To those who might struggle with this message

I've spent many hours thinking about some of the people I know, many of whom are also Christians, and their possible reactions to this book. I know that some consider Eastern meditation practices "un-Godly," but I still feel compelled to try to give these good people some new options for thought in the only way I know how.

And that way is by sharing my own personal experiences. In the previous story, my wife and I, skeptics both, set aside our skepticism just long enough to open ourselves to the possibility that there might be something for us to learn. And there was.

In the same way I had discovered many years ago that chiropractic is as viable as other medical practices, and in the same way I am now discovering more and more methods to help people achieve good health that are outside the purely conventional, I am also discovering that "alternative" methods for practicing spirituality do nothing but *enhance* what we already know.

Just as there are alternative medical techniques, there are alternative religious or spiritual ones. None of the alternative medical treatments are there to blot out Western medicine and, in the same way, practicing meditative techniques as a complement to Christian belief (or any other form of religious belief) does not negate or take away from one's heartfelt religion. In other words, it's not about leaving one behind for the other; it's about adding another tool to your toolbox of communing with God (or whatever name you choose to call your Source and Savior).

It seems to me that to live in the spirit of Christ, to act in the ways He would have us act, is to connect with God as much as possible, to try to make ourselves more "whole" and "balanced" in the way we live our lives. To me, this includes the way we approach our health because our health is affected by our beliefs, our stress levels, our attitudes, and our ability to see beyond what is right in front of us.

Addressing the whole

All religions have one thing in common: a belief in the "Christ element"—a belief that we should all try to achieve wholeness.

It is when we are elevated out of a place of consciousness—the place of trials and tribulations we all know so well—that we understand our elevation is due to that element of Christ that we have been fortunate to experience. Giving ourselves opportunities to experience a relief from trials and tribulations related to poor health is one significant way to improve the relationship we have with our God.

We do not have to feel that mediation detracts from our prayers or our devotion. In fact, meditation brings with it a kind of stress relief that allows us to pray with even more openness and thankfulness. When I looked up "meditation" in the dictionary, I read two definitions: (1) *continued or extended thought; reflection; contemplation* and (2) *devout religious contemplation or spiritual introspection*, and was surprised by the lack of any meaning that would imply that meditation was in opposition to any kind of religious practices. In fact, "devout religious contemplation" *is* meditation.

So where's the rub?

The rub comes when we define our practices so rigidly that we forget the nature of what we want to accomplish.

The AMA has done this year after year by forgetting that its primary goal as a group of physicians is to heal.

The drug companies do this by forgetting to place people over profits.

And we forget that in order to achieve health and balance and a sense of wholeness, we need to let go of rigidity and stay open to exploration—even as we live devout lives.

As a devout Christian, I can only say that far from leading me astray, meditating has actually led me closer to understanding myself, my universe, and God.

If I can encourage even one person to explore new realms of consciousness to help him or her achieve a higher state of health and balance, I will have reached my ultimate goal.

CHAPTER EIGHTEEN

APPLYING WHAT I'VE LEARNED

An interesting thing happened two years ago. I had a dream (actually, there was a voice) that I remembered when I woke up and it was so clear, so powerful that I needed to tell my wife. As I got out of bed, very groggy, I thought, "If I still remember this dream this evening, I'll share it with her." I usually don't remember my dreams.

The evening came, and I hadn't forgotten. As we were getting ready for bed, I said, "Janice, I had a dream last night only it wasn't visual, it was auditory. You're going to think it's off the wall, but I want to tell you. My dream was a distinct, clear, commanding voice that said, 'You need to go to Barcelona.'"

She asked if it gave any indication of when. I responded, "I don't know." She asked why. I responded, "I don't know." I told her it was so powerful that it felt like a message from God.

Since there was no timeframe given, we didn't rush to make any plans. We both agreed that we would get additional signs or messages directing us when the time was right.

Two years went by and our ten-year anniversary was approaching, so we needed to plan a special trip for this milestone in our lives together. We discussed different options: maybe Hawaii, maybe wine country... Then we both looked at each other, smiled and practically at the same time said, "Barcelona." We immediately began searching for flights and hotels, and making plans.

The time finally came for our trip. I was somewhat pensive,

wondering if we made the right decision that would let us have the best time possible on this important occasion. On the other hand, I worried that I wouldn't find my purpose or discover why I even had the dream in the first place. After all, prior to and since then, I've never had a dream direct me to do something.

Our flight to Spain was fantastic. For our first three days there, we rented a car and would get off the freeway at random exits just for the heck of it. There were no rules, no deadlines, no cell phones or computers. We met wonderful people, had wonderful food and saw places we would have never seen had we been on a tour bus going from point A to B. Each day got better and better, and made us realize that we were doing things too hard in the U.S. Everyone in Spain seemed to take life a bit less seriously and there was a very positive vibe everywhere we went. We were constantly in great moods.

As our trip continued, we decided to go to Montserrat, a holy mountain and monastery (which is cited in many places as one of the greatest religious shrines in Spain). I had a feeling that this would be where I found an answer for the dream I had two years ago.

We took a train from Barcelona to Montserrat; I'll never forget the spectacular view of the tan mountains that rose up out of a relatively flat terrain. We took another train that wrapped around the mountain, going all the way to the monastery. When we arrived, I walked around, praying, asking God if He would direct me to something that might explain why I had my dream.

We walked into the monastery, where we stood in line to touch the statue of the Madonna and Child, which is said to bring blessings and miracles. It was quite an amazing sight: parents brought infants up and laid their babies' hands on the statue; adults said a short prayer as they touched the figures, as did I. Although the monastery was beautiful, I hadn't received any answers or signs.

Coming out, we realized there was another peak reachable by a funicular, a railway car that gets pulled up a very steep incline by a cable. We made it to the top of that mountain and began to walk on a wide path where people were taking photos and checking out the view.

Now may be a good time to mention my fear of heights. I have a paralyzing fear when I'm up high and not enclosed in some type of vehicle. Still, I was doing pretty well so far. As we walked, we came to a waist-high ledge leading to a narrow path that went up about 300 more feet to the peak. Suddenly, I heard a voice in my mind that told me to go up and find some special rocks to take back to my children from this holy place.

I didn't say anything to Janice about the voice; I just told her that I was going to go up to get some rocks for the kids. Knowing my fear of heights, she asked me to please be careful. I hopped up on the ledge then crouched down to look for rocks. Then I heard the voice say, "Go farther."

I began walking this dirt path that was about two feet wide with knee-high bushes on both sides. I was going slowly and shaking because the higher I went, the more I could see of the surrounding plains 4,000 feet below. After walking 50 feet, scared and breathing heavily, I squatted down and said, "OK, God, this is a beautiful place. I'm going to find some great rocks for my kids here." The voice answered, "Go farther."

I sighed, terrified to go any farther. Slowly I got up, my hands and knees shaking, and began to walk some more, about 25 feet. I stopped and thought, *This is plenty*, then squatted down, nearly having an anxiety attack, to look for rocks. Again I heard, "Go farther."

I said, "God, this is Your plan. I trust You and Your Word." Interestingly, I stood up and walked, then walked faster, then *ran*. I had no fear, no anxiety, no shaking. I kept repeating, "I trust you, God" over and over until I finally made it to the top. The view was incredible! Although I could no longer see Janice where she was standing, I felt empowered and liberated for overcoming my paralyzing acrophobia.

I picked up a few special rocks then just stood there, with the wind blowing powerfully at the peak. I heard the same voice, only this time it said something different: "You didn't come up to the top to find rocks…that's how I got you here. The lesson is that, with your book, you will face adversity from some critics but people need to hear what you have to say regarding health. By facing and conquering your biggest fear, you have proven that you're ready to face any adversity. Just deliver the message."

I continued listening in amazement as the message kept coming: "Whatever good or bad happens in your life, you must understand that the reason for it is My Will. Don't look at negative things as something bad. Both negative and positive will happen to you; do not react with extreme emotion. Understand that it's happening for a reason—to teach you the lessons that will lead you down the path I have chosen for you."

This was the most unbelievably spiritual moment I have ever experienced in my life. For all the times I asked God to give me a sign or said a prayer and never got an immediate answer, this was spectacular! I just sat there in awe, thinking about all the things that I had considered negative or adverse: flights I missed because of traffic on the way to the airport, long lines at the grocery store that "inconvenienced" me. I thought, *What if those were all times when God was setting me up to serve or help someone who needed assistance in some way, and I missed the opportunity?* Maybe I should have accepted that that was the way things were meant to be and struck up a conversation with the person behind me in line instead of being angry and irritable.

I declared right then that things would change in my life. Although I thought I was doing things right, I could have been doing them better.

When I made my way down the mountain trail back to Janice, I told her bits and pieces of the enlightening experience. I couldn't contain my excitement—and I held out my hand and said, "You have to come see the beautiful view and the place where this epiphany occurred." She was afraid to step up on the ledge but I said, "Janice, God spoke directly to me. Please share this experience. It won't be complete unless you come to the top with me."

She agreed but walked cautiously and slowly; I was pulling her along because of my enthusiasm and sudden lack of acrophobia. We made it to the top and Janice couldn't believe the view. The wind was blowing so hard that it was difficult to hear each other, so we sat down and I further explained the rest of my recent experience, speaking closely into her ear. When I finished the story, the wind stopped—it literally went from tropical storm speeds to absolutely nothing, not even a slight breeze. Neither one of us said a word or moved a muscle for about two minutes. It was such a solemn, spiritual experience.

The trip to Spain felt complete. I broke the silence by asking quietly, "Can you believe that?" Janice responded by shaking her head slightly, her eyes wide open.

We both felt recharged and I said a prayer, "God, I think I'll be ready for the path that You have chosen for me. Thank You for such an unbelievable experience."

I was put to the test the following day, to see if I really did learn something. After a fun dinner with great food, a bottle of wine and fantastic conversation, we took a taxi back to the hotel. We were toting a bunch of bags, camera cases, etc., which we grabbed after I paid the driver. After making our way up to our room and putting everything down, I emptied my pockets and my heart stopped for a second. My wallet wasn't there!

I told Janice and her heart skipped a beat as well. That wallet had our drivers' licenses, the majority of our cash, all my credit cards, health insurance cards, auto insurance cards, and a very special piece of paper with a prayer my Grandmother wrote, which I found among her things a few days after she passed.

I ran downstairs frantically and told the hotel staff. Since I didn't have the taxi number, it would be virtually impossible to track it down; it had left already left 10 minutes before. I called the U.S. to cancel my credit cards then had American Express wire some money. In the middle of all this, I said to Janice, "Wait a second. This is one of the tests, the 'chosen path' I learned of at the top of the mountain. We can't react emotionally to this…it is what it is."

I reasoned that the credit cards were just plastic, the money was just paper and my Grandmother's prayer had already guided her and me. I suddenly found myself saying, "Oh, well, it's just a wallet," then turned to Janice and said, "Tomorrow's our last day in Spain. Let's make it a great one."

Prior to my experience at Montserrat, I would have been an emotional wreck, pacing the floor, thinking about what I had lost and about every negative outcome that could possibly happen. I was okay with things, though. I realized how much we all let stress affect us and make us miss out on really important moments—and it's usually just due to overreacting about material things. Stress kills and I knew we all needed to learn to make every attempt to eliminate it from our lives. Many people say that when they have stress, they leave it in God's hands. Yet they continue to get upset over the same things to the point where they develop anxiety disorders. It's easy to say that you let go of your problems, but tough to do.

As far as losing my wallet, I really did leave it in God's hands—and the last day of our trip wasn't stressful at all. With no wallet, credit cards or cash in my pocket, I looked into my wife's eyes, smiled and kissed her, realizing how much I really did have. I said, "This was a fantastic ten-year anniversary. I love you."

When we made it home, I told Janice not to say anything about the missing wallet to anyone. Most people unknowingly gravitate toward the negative and I knew we'd get more questions about the wallet than about all of the awesome things we did and saw in Spain. That would just bring us down and cast a shadow on our trip. We told very few people and, amazingly, not discussing it allowed us to simply put the one negative thing behind us and move on, focusing on our family, friends and, of course, my patients.

And that lesson is the one I would most like to pass on to you.

Remember, lighten up, life's problems are only as big as YOU make them. Problems are just part of God's lessons and are merely opportunities for us to grow, both mentally and spiritually. It's time to begin to change your viewpoints on healthcare so you can live a more productive life. Let the first step be allowing your brain to function like a parachute; it works a whole lot better when it's open.

INDEX

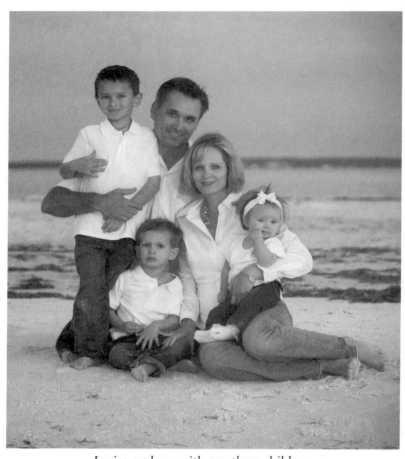

Janice and me with our three children,
Tyler, Nicholas and Hannah Rose.